The Church and AIDS in Africa

The Church and AIDS in Africa

The Politics of Ambiguity

Amy S. Patterson

FIRSTFORUMPRESS

A DIVISION OF LYNNE RIENNER PUBLISHERS, INC. • BOULDER & LONDON

Published in the United States of America in 2011 by
FirstForumPress
A division of Lynne Rienner Publishers, Inc.
1800 30th Street, Boulder, Colorado 80301
www.firstforumpress.com

and in the United Kingdom by
FirstForumPress
A division of Lynne Rienner Publishers, Inc.
3 Henrietta Street, Covent Garden, London WC2E 8LU

Library of Congress Cataloging-in-Publication Data
A Cataloging-in-Publication record for this book
is available from the Library of Congress.
ISBN: 978-1-935049-04-3

British Cataloguing in Publication Data
A Cataloguing in Publication record for this book
is available from the British Library.

This book was produced from digital files
prepared using the FirstForumComposer.

Printed and bound in the United States of America

The paper used in this publication meets the requirements
of the American National Standard for Permanence of
Paper for Printed Library Materials Z39.48-1992.

5 4 3 2 1

To five young women,
two girls,
and one good-natured man…

zikomo, medasi, weebale, xie xie, jërëjëf, thank you

Contents

Tables and Figures

Tables

Figures

Acknowledgments

While I was finishing this manuscript, I was honored with a college-wide teaching award for advising and mentoring students. After I received the news about the honor from my dean, I thought about how ironic the award was, particularly in light of this project. For it was my students who pushed, prodded, and questioned me; who read, searched, and endured alongside me; and who, ultimately, made this book possible.

Five young women—all former Calvin students—deserve special thanks. Kyla Vander Hart travelled with me to Zambia for research in 2007. Not only did she keep me from missing flights as I dozed during long airport layovers, but she also put up with my demands. Even though her first trip to Africa at times overwhelmed and exhausted her, she smiled as she set up interviews, typed data, and hung out with her college professor for several weeks. During fall 2008, Becky Bouman and Katie Sytsema scheduled and accompanied me on interviews in Accra, Ghana. As part of the Calvin College Off-Campus Semester Program, they went above and beyond the requirements of their independent study. Not only did they hold their breath and cover their eyes as I drove in the Accra traffic (sometimes the goal for the day was merely to get to the interview without an accident), but their questions helped me to process what we learned. To Emily Keller, I owe many thanks for happily indexing Ghana interviews and finding additional research materials. And I have unending gratitude for Michelle Fraser, who read and reread the manuscript, found and updated statistics, posed questions, listened to my endless "thinking out loud," and noticed all my typos. Not only did she help greatly with this project, but she also did invaluable work for a 2010 Uganda workshop on AIDS, religion, and social activism that I helped to organize.

More broadly, after more than a dozen years of teaching, my students continue to encourage and inspire me. Their honest questions, particularly those queries from participants in the 2008 Calvin College semester in Ghana program, demand answers. As I seek to meet their challenges, I hope I have become not only a better teacher and researcher, but also a better person.

Many people made research in Zambia and Ghana possible in 2007, 2008, and 2009. The staff at Justo Mwale Theological College in Lusaka helped me with logistical arrangements during my 2007 stay. African pastors and seminary professors associated with the Network for African Congregational Theology (NETACT) welcomed my questions at a 2007 conference and enlightened me on the challenges they faced in addressing AIDS and poverty. In particular, I thank Jurgens Hendriks (Stellenbosch University) for making the 2007 NETACT conference possible and Corwin Smidt (Calvin College) for urging me to participate. In Ghana, I owe special thanks to Ben and Awo Asiedu for making my months in Accra enjoyable. Laura McGough at the University of Ghana and Valerie Gueye at the Willows Foundation helped me to better understand some of my observations. I wish to thank the numerous pastors, AIDS activists, leaders of faith-based organizations, scholars, leaders of ecumenical associations, government representatives, and donor officials in Africa and the United States for participating in interviews and patiently answering my questions.

The International Research Network on Religion and AIDS in Africa, particularly Marian Burchardt, Hansjörg Dilger, Alessandro Gusman, Louise Rasmussen, and Rijk van Dijk, provided support and creative ideas throughout this and related projects. Participants in the 2010 summer workshop on AIDS, religion, and social activism held at the Child Health and Development Centre, Makerere University, also sharpened my thinking. I am grateful to two anonymous reviewers for their insights on the manuscript.

No project is possible without time, opportunities, and money. Calvin College has generously provided all three. Travel to Zambia was made possible through grants from the Alumni Association and the Provost's Office. The Nagel Institute for the Study of World Christianity partially supported travel to Zambia in 2009, and the Calvin Center for Christian Scholarship funded the summer 2010 workshop in Uganda on AIDS, religion, and social activism. My involvement with the 2010 project pushed me to further delve into the nuances of church mobilization on AIDS and to make important connections to other scholars working on the topic. I wish to thank the Calvin College administration and the Board of Trustees for a sabbatical leave, course releases through the Calvin Research Fellowship program, and an interim leave to complete research and writing. The McGregor program and the Paul Henry Institute funded student assistants for several years. And the Calvin College Off-Campus Semester Program made my stay in Ghana possible, an opportunity that not only facilitated this research but also allowed my family to live and learn in Africa.

I couldn't have better colleagues: Joel Carpenter, Roland Hoksbergen, Doug Koopman, Tracy Kuperus, and Mwenda Ntarangwi read parts of the work, gave me methodological insights, and urged me to get the project done. Ellen Hekman proofread, while Joyce Steigenga helped with computer issues. Two Calvin Center for Christian Scholarship reading groups—one on African Christianity and the other on global health—helped me to think more clearly about the interview findings, as did the Calvin College–sponsored 2009 summer colloquium on the social implications of African Christianity. I remain grateful that I can work *and learn* in such a supportive and challenging environment.

Two girls and their good-natured father make my life complete. Thank you Isabel, Sophia, and Neil, for smiling, laughing, traveling to Africa, wanting to learn more, and caring about the project and, more important, the continent's people. I love you longer than the Great Wall, more vibrant than the colors in Asante *kente* cloth, and deeper than the well in Santiou Ndioubene, Senegal.

1
AIDS and Christianity in Africa

Churches in sub-Saharan Africa have been maligned, vilified, praised, and ignored for their role in the fight against the Acquired Immunodeficiency Syndrome (AIDS). Such divergent reactions from scholars, activists, and development officials are unsurprising given the diversity of church responses to the pandemic.[1] Contrast the public statement of Dr. Kwesi Dickson, former general secretary of the All Africa Conference of Churches, with that of Bishop Boniface Setlalekgosi, head of the Catholic Church in Botswana. In a 2003 speech, Dickson placed AIDS in the larger context of poverty, poor governance, and underdevelopment in Africa. He demanded that both governments and churches pay greater attention to the Africans whose lives were being decimated by poverty and disease (*AACC Newsletter*, November 25, 2003). Conversely, Bishop Setlalekgosi took a more narrow approach, portraying AIDS as a question of individual morality. He wrote in a 2004 letter to youth: "Unfortunately, you are … flooded with wrong messages that give false security, that of 'condomise and stay alive'" (*Mgegi/The Reporter*, August 6, 2004).

Or compare the actions of Prophetess Lucy Nduta of the Nairobi-based Salvation Healing Church with those of congregants in a Cape Town Baptist church. The prophetess insisted that she cured her followers of the Human Immunodeficiency Virus (HIV), the virus that causes AIDS, through prayer and healing services (*Nation*, May 22, 2006). Her actions illustrated her belief in the power of the invisible, spiritual realm to overcome the physical world's problems. In contrast to her spiritual approach, the formation by South African Baptists of the Living Hope Community Centre was rooted in the physical world. The Baptist congregants responded to the immediate physical needs of people living with HIV/AIDS because of their conviction that a combination of physical and spiritual support can improve quality of life.[2]

These four examples illustrate points along the spectrum of church responses to AIDS. While they could be studied as contrasting models of service provision or as the embodiment of theology in practice, my interest in them is in their political nature. Politics is the process of decision-making that shapes resource allocation and acceptance of particular values. Politics occurs in formal arenas, such as legislatures, election campaigns, and bureaucracies, but it also exists in civil society organizations, families, and the workplace. The above-mentioned church actions directly or indirectly challenge power structures in society, and they seek to affect decisions about resource allocation and the acceptance of certain values. When Dickson challenged governments on the relationship between AIDS and poverty, when Bishop Setlalekgosi and Prophetess Nduta used faith to point to powers beyond science, and when the Baptists reached out to marginalized members of society, they all engaged in politics.

At times the AIDS activities that are discussed in this book do not look political. What is political about caring for someone who is dying from AIDS or about urging youth to abstain from sex? I argue that there is something "subversive" about these actions (Miller and Yamamori 2007, 5); they sometimes challenge the established science on AIDS or the donor community's policies; they question the ability of the state to meet its end of the social contract; and they defy global and national-level political and economic structures that often downplay the human rights and dignity of poor Africans. In so doing, many churches are engaging in a form of social activism, or a process by which they challenge the status quo in their churches, communities, countries, and/or the international realm.

The currency of such political activism is power. Power can be rooted in tangible elements, like government authority, material resources, large constituencies, expertise, and tools of physical coercion. Dickson and the All Africa Conference of Churches have some of this tangible power, since the organization counts as members 169 churches, church councils, and theological institutions in forty countries, and it represents more than 120 million African Christians (AACC 2008). But power is also located in intangible sources such as moral authority, symbols, and, for many Africans, the spiritual realm. The Catholic bishop's letter relies on his moral authority, and the prophetess who claims to cure HIV taps into the idea that "spiritual belief offers access to an alternative form of power" (Ellis and ter Haar 1998, 195). Symbolic metaphors rooted in religious imagery or texts may either mobilize or demobilize participation in AIDS efforts (see Vander Meulen 2010). Unlike Western liberalism, African conceptions of politics and religion do not divide the sacred and the secular. Even if formal constitutions outline a secular state, political life is often "inextricably bound up with religious belief" (Jenkins 2007, 162). The public and private actions of churches themselves influence politics (VonDoepp 1998). While my focus is on Christian majority states, this is also true in countries with large Muslim majorities, as Muslim leaders' long-time involvement in elections in Senegal illustrates (Villalón 1995).

Just as has been the case with secular efforts to address AIDS, religiously based responses involve contentious processes of identity formation and frame alignment. Religious adherents have struggled both among themselves and in relation to secular activists to define a common identity that drives their involvement on AIDS. While some religious actors involved with AIDS are HIV-positive, this is not the case for all participants. What identity then facilitates action? The development of a unifying identity to propel activities is a process shaped by power, representation, and constructs of ideas (Melucci 1996). Similarly, the process of framing the AIDS issue may include some, while excluding others. For example, when AIDS is framed as an issue that primarily affects innocent women and children, then HIV-positive men are excluded from potential policy outcomes or mobilization efforts. The way the issue is understood affects who gets access to resources and power (Snow et al. 1986); such processes occur in religious institutions just as they do in secular groups.

In this book, I use the word *church* broadly, to mean both an institution and a community of individual believers. Institutionally, church congregations and denominations have rules, formal and informal norms, officials, material resources, and histories (North 1990, 3). My institutional definition includes church-related organizations like health care facilities, advocacy wings, ecumenical networks, and centers of theological education. The process of church institutionalization occurs over time, with newer churches often lacking the formal bodies, rules, well-defined liturgy, and specialized leadership training of the churches established by the colonial missionaries. The church is also a fluid and diverse community of individuals who identify themselves as Christian and who believe the biblical messages of Christianity. Newer churches may lack well-defined institutions, but they do not lack the fervor of belief among their members (Jenkins 2007, 157-158). While I do examine church leaders as instigators of AIDS programs, my general focus is on churches as institutions, not on individual Christian believers.

In the pages that follow, I analyze the interactions between churches—as institutions and as communities of believers—and politics on the AIDS issue. These interactions take on various forms, and these forms often are not mutually exclusive. To be clear, I do not argue for more or less church involvement in the political questions surrounding AIDS. The church's role on AIDS is controversial, both within Christian circles and between Christians and non-Christians. In the Western experience, particularly during the first years of the AIDS epidemic, the church was viewed as an obstacle to AIDS efforts. Many AIDS organizations were secular, often organized by HIV-positive gay men and their HIV-negative friends or partners. The regular protests of ACT UP–New York in front of St. Patrick's Cathedral demonstrate this tension. But the situation in Africa has been different, because many members of AIDS groups (both the majority who are HIV-positive and their HIV-negative supporters) are religious believers; they may be church members who regularly attend services, pray daily, and read the Bible. This African reality complicates church mobilization against AIDS and challenges assumptions that religion and activism cannot coexist (Siplon 2010; Dilger 2010).

This book is not intended to be a theological treatise or a defense of or challenge to Christian belief. Rather, I acknowledge that religion is important for a large number of Africans, and as such, cannot be ignored in any analysis of social, political, or economic issues. What I seek to do is to move beyond the tendency to portray churches as either stigmatizing obstacles or charity do-gooders (Dilger 2007, 59). Churches play a complicated role in the AIDS pandemic because of their diverse historical experiences, resources, leadership styles, and theological perspectives. This variation leads to different forms of mobilization and ways to frame the AIDS issue. My assumptions about churches' responses to AIDS were sometimes challenged during the course of the research: churches that I did not think would respond to AIDS had well-developed programs; churches that I thought would be progressive in dealing with AIDS-related issues (such as gender equality or condom distribution) were not. Church interviewees I least expected to be compassionate in the struggle with AIDS told compelling stories of church efforts, while those I most expected to care about the issue dismissed my questions.

What became clear through the research was that making blanket statements about churches and AIDS responses, as both church critics and advocates tend to do, does not contribute to an analysis of church mobilization on the AIDS issue. On the other hand, because social scientists recognize that some generalizations are helpful for examining patterns of behavior or institutional structures, I set up a five-fold typology of church responses based on the timing and breadth of church AIDS actions: (1) no response; (2) the early, narrow response; (3) the early, broad response; (4) the late, narrow response; and (5) the late, broad response. This model may not initially be intuitive, particularly for readers with strong views on specific AIDS policies, such as condom distribution, abstinence-only education, or HIV prevention efforts to men who have sex with men. As I explain in Chapter 2, rather than narrow my analysis to the substance of one or two policies to classify mobilization patterns, I analyze a wide variety of church responses and the complex reasons for those actions. Given the often dynamic and multi-faceted AIDS activities of many churches, the model provides a more accurate picture of church actions on the ground. Chapter 2 fully defines the model and gives examples. The rest of the book uses explanations based on resources, organizational structures, relations with the state, and global networks to elucidate why churches have fallen into one of the five patterns.

Africa is a religiously plural continent. Even though an estimated 57 percent of people in sub-Saharan Africa are Christian, 29 percent are Muslims and 13 percent practice African traditional religions. When one compares Islam and Christianity across all of Africa, the numbers are much closer, but because North Africa has unique historical experiences, political and socioeconomic linkages to the Middle East, and a predominantly Arab culture, I only focus on sub-Saharan Africa. Surveys and ethnographies further illustrate that adherence to Christianity or Islam south of the Sahara does not necessarily exclude individual involvement in African traditional religious practices, such as the use of diviners or healers. While I acknowledge this complexity, the book limits its scope to focus on Christian responses to AIDS. In Chapters 3 and 5, however, I incorporate analysis of how those church responses have shaped church relations with Muslim and African traditional religious institutions and leaders. This analysis is situated in a context where Muslim-Christian tensions have increased over the last decade, particularly in light of religiously based violence (Pew Forum 2010).

Church AIDS activities occur on a continent where Christianity is growing, many civil society groups play a political and economic role, and bilateral and multilateral donors have given large amounts of funding to faith-based organizations to fight AIDS. To explicate this context, I first provide background on Africa's AIDS pandemic. Next, in order to comprehend how churches differ in their AIDS approaches, I describe the growth of Christianity in Africa and distinguish various types of churches. Because churches are often defined as civil society organizations, the chapter investigates how adequately the civil society paradigm applies to religious organizations in African politics. Finally, I highlight recent bilateral and multilateral donor attention to churches and AIDS. Increased funding and recognition give these religious bodies a greater stake in AIDS and necessitate that political scientists, donors, and activists more thoroughly investigate their role in AIDS politics.

African Churches Confront AIDS

Churches have numerous reasons to be concerned about AIDS. The first, and most obvious, is the magnitude of the pandemic. In 2005, the Joint United Nations Program on HIV/AIDS (UNAIDS), the agency that coordinates all United Nations activities on AIDS, predicted that without continued large-scale commitment to fight AIDS, eighty million Africans would die from the disease by 2025 (UNAIDS 2005a, 110). While AIDS is a global problem, sub-Saharan Africa has been particularly hard hit. The region has over two-thirds of the world's thirty-three million people infected with HIV. In 2008, 1.4 million Africans died from AIDS (UNAIDS 2009a).

In reality, AIDS affects African countries differently, with each experiencing its own unique epidemic. HIV epidemics are classified into four types: (1) low-level epidemic; (2) concentrated epidemic; (3) generalized low-level epidemic; and (4) generalized high-level epidemic. In low-level epidemics, HIV prevalence is below 1 percent in the general population and less than 5 percent in key populations with greater HIV infection risks. These most-at-risk groups include commercial sex workers, men who have sex with men, and intravenous drug users. Because HIV tends to be transmitted heterosexually or from mother-to-child during pregnancy, delivery, or breastfeeding in Africa, epidemiologists often rely on HIV prevalence in the general population to classify a country's epidemic. Also, it is difficult to get accurate data on HIV in key populations such as sex workers or men who have sex with men because of the often illegal and stigmatized nature of their activities. For these reasons, I classify epidemics based on prevalence levels in the general population in Tables 1.1 and 1.2.

In the concentrated, generalized low-level, and generalized high-level epidemics, HIV prevalence in key populations is more than 5 percent, although prevalence in the general population differs. In a concentrated epidemic, as found in Senegal and Somalia, less than 1 percent of the general population is HIV positive. In a generalized, low-level epidemic such as in Ghana, Eritrea, and Kenya, HIV prevalence in the general population is between 1 and 10 percent. Countries with generalized high-level epidemics, such as Zambia, South Africa, and Namibia, have general prevalence rates that are 10 percent or more. Some of the most extreme generalized, high-level epidemics are in the southern African countries of Botswana, Lesotho, Swaziland, and Zimbabwe, where prevalence rates are above 20 percent (UNAIDS 2009a; UCSF 2008).

Beyond the magnitude of the pandemic, churches are interested in AIDS because the Bible commands believers to care for the sick. In Matthew 25:31-46, Christ tells his followers that caring for the sick, lonely, imprisoned, and naked is the same as caring for him. One cannot love Christ and ignore the "least of these" in society. Christ himself heals those with physical ailments (the paralyzed, the bleeding woman, the leper, and the blind), demonstrating the importance of both physical and spiritual health and illustrating that the two are linked.[3] Other biblical passages urge believers to care for widows and orphans, and to love and accept society's most vulnerable members, such as children.[4] While not all churches emphasize these messages, they are key Christian teachings. In Chapter 3, I examine divergent biblical understandings of AIDS as one explanation for why churches have adopted different patterns in their AIDS responses.

Churches also are concerned about AIDS because African citizens are increasingly prioritizing the disease as a public issue. The Kaiser Foundation and Pew Forum found that in seven of ten countries surveyed in 2007, citizens ranked "AIDS and other diseases" as the biggest problem their country faces.[5] In South Africa, 88 percent of respondents ranked AIDS and other diseases as a big problem, second only to crime. Even in Nigeria and Mali where the issue was ranked as the third biggest problem, over 60 percent of respondents mentioned it (Kaiser Family Foundation and Pew Forum 2007). While the survey does not give information on the intensity of these opinions, it does demonstrate public concern about health, including AIDS.

The magnitude of AIDS, biblical messages, and growing concern in society about health are compelling reasons for churches to react to AIDS. Church leaders often add to this list when they assert that as an institution rooted in society, the church cannot ignore the various impacts of AIDS (Interviews 9, 10).[6] For example, life expectancy has fallen by almost five years in Africa, both because of AIDS and because HIV infections make individuals more vulnerable to death from other diseases such as malaria and tuberculosis (*Business Day*, June 20, 2006). Churches are aware of the negative effects of AIDS on education, health care, and businesses. In Mozambique, for example, one-sixth of the country's teachers die annually of AIDS-related causes (*Reuters*, March 25, 2008). Similarly, Gold Fields, one of the world's largest gold producers, estimates that the total cost of HIV infections is around $5 per ounce of gold mined in South Africa (*Reuters*, July 11, 2007). And churches have had to directly confront the fact that twelve million African children have lost one or both parents to AIDS (AVERT 2008). Churches recognize that not only do many of these children lose material support, but they also lose love, guidance, and nurturing.

Beyond these social, theological, and economic reasons, churches have found it increasingly difficult to ignore AIDS because, as one church official remarked, "The church has AIDS" (Interview 2). Pastors, lay leaders, and congregants are HIV positive, and millions of African Christians have died from AIDS. The church has not been spared the personal, family, and societal effects of the disease; one South African pastor remarked, "We are overwhelmed."[7] Yet, it would be simplistic and cynical to view church concern over AIDS as purely instrumental. One Zambian church official explained, "We care for people because they are hurting and dying, not because of their religion" (Interview 17). Another religious leader said that even in countries with low-level epidemics and small Christian populations, the church is concerned about all people's health (Interview 53).

While the church proclaims concern for all people living with HIV/AIDS, one cannot deny that the disease has greatly affected countries with large Christian populations. Table 1.1 provides data on religious percentages and HIV prevalence rates for most of the forty-eight countries in sub-Saharan Africa. The table relies on the *World Christian Encyclopedia*, which is compiled for 238 countries by 450 global experts. However, getting reliable data on religion is problematic. One challenge is definitions: Are "Christians" people who attend church or individuals who profess belief? Here I follow Philip Jenkins' model (2007, 102) and define Christians as professing believers, not church attendees. Governments also may have an interest in shaping religious data, and religious groups may dispute census results (Jenkins 2007, 100-105; 190-192).[8] While I acknowledge these (and other) data challenges, I use the statistics to demonstrate general trends, not to give exact numbers of religious adherents.

Table 1.1 indicates that Christianity is the majority religion in twenty-six countries; Islam, in eleven; and ethno-religions (or traditional religions), in two. There is no majority religion in nine countries, although Christians compose at least one-third (33 percent) of the population in four of those nine. Muslim-majority countries are primarily in the Horn of Africa and West Africa, while Christian-dominated countries tend to be in southern, eastern, and central Africa.

In terms of HIV prevalence and a country's majority religion, the mean HIV prevalence for countries with a Christian majority (excluding Cape Verde, Sao Tome and Principe, and Seychelles, for which there is no HIV data) is 9.5 percent. For Muslim countries, the mean HIVrate is 1.39 percent. For countries with no religious majority, it is 2.14 percent. Because there are only two with majority ethno-religionists, and their HIV rates are far apart (Mozambique's is 12.5% and Benin's is 1.2%), the mean for these two countries—6.85 percent—does not provide much information. The most apparent trend of this data is that the mean HIV rate for Christian majority countries is much higher than it is for Muslim majority countries.

Table 1.2 provides another picture of the relationship between epidemic type and majority religion. The table divides countries based on epidemic types and majority religion. It shows that 57.6 percent of Christian-majority countries have generalized low-level epidemics and 30.7 percent have generalized high-level epidemics. In contrast, 54.5 percent of Muslim-majority countries have a generalized, low-level epidemic and 45.4 percent have a concentrated epidemic. Of the thirty countries with a generalized low-level epidemic, fifteen are Christian majority, six are Muslim majority, one is majority ethno-religious, and eight are religiously plural. However, the correlation between Christian majority and HIV prevalence is most evident in high-level epidemic countries. Of the nine countries with generalized high-level epidemics, eight are majority Christian. The other, Mozambique, has an ethno-religionist majority and a sizeable Christian minority.

While the data provide some general patterns about the relationship between HIV prevalence and religious majority, they are limited by the small number of cases, particularly for countries with an ethno-religionist majority. Although the data say nothing about causality between religious dominance and HIV prevalence, scholars have put forward some explanations based on economic structures and religious and cultural practices for the Muslim-Christian pattern found in Table 1.2. The economic structure of southern Africa, a region with generalized, high-level epidemics and large Christian populations, has encouraged high rates of labor migration. Mines in South Africa, Zambia, and Botswana have attracted millions of workers, many of whom spend long periods away from home. Migrants are more likely to have multiple sexual partners, providing greater opportunity for HIV to spread rapidly (Campbell 2003, 28-35; Barnett and Whiteside 2002, 87, 122).

Table 1.1 Religion, HIV Prevalence, and Epidemic Type, by Country

Country	Christian (2000)	Muslim (2000)	Ethno-religion[a] (2000)	Other[b] (2000)	No Religion[c] (2000)	HIV Prevalence[d] (2007)	Epidemic Type
Angola	94.1		5.0	1	0.5	2.1	generalized, low level
Benin	28.5	20	51.5	0.5		1.2	generalized, low level
Botswana	59.9	0.2	38.8	1		23.9	generalized, high level
Burkina Faso	16.7	48.6	34.2		1	2.0	generalized, low level
Burundi	91.7	1.4	6.7	0.5		3.3	generalized, low level
Cameroon	54.2	21.2	23.7	1		5.1	generalized, low level
Cape Verde	95.1	2.8	1.1	1		no data[e]	
Central African Republic	67.8	15.8	15.4	1	1	6.3	generalized, low level
Chad	22.8	59.1	17	1		3.5	generalized, low level
Comoros	1.2	98		<1	<1	<0.1	concentrated
Congo-Brazzaville	91.2	1.3	4.8	1	2	3.5	generalized, low level
Côte d'Ivoire	31.8	30.1	37.6	<0.5	<0.5	3.9	generalized, low level
Democratic Republic of Congo	95.4	1.1	2.4	0.5	0.5	3.2[f]	generalized, low level
Djibouti	4.5	94.1		<1	1.3	3.1	generalized, low level
Equatorial Guinea	88.4	4.1	2.1	<1	~5.0	3.4	generalized, low level
Eritrea	50.5	44.7	0.6		4.1	1.3	generalized, low level
Ethiopia	57.7	30.4	11.7		<0.5	2.1	generalized, low level
Gabon	90.6	4.6	3.1	0.5	1	5.9	generalized, low level
Gambia	3.9	86.9	7.8	~1.0	<0.5	0.9	concentrated
Ghana	55.4	19.7	24.4	<0.5	<0.5	1.9	generalized, low level
Guinea	4.0	67.8	28.5		<0.5	1.6	generalized, low level
Guinea-Bissau	13.2	39	45.2		1.5	1.8	generalized, low level
Kenya	79.3	7.3	11.5	<2	<0.5	7.1-8.5[g]	generalized, low level
Lesotho	91.0	0.1	7.7	~1		23.2	generalized, high level
Liberia	39.3	16	42.9	<0.5	1.5	1.7	generalized, low level
Madagascar	49.5	2.0	48	<0.5	<0.5	0.1	concentrated[h]
Malawi	76.8	14.8	7.8	<0.5	<0.5	11.9	generalized, high level
Mali	2.0	81.9	16			1.5	generalized, low level
Mauritania	0.3	99.1	0.5			0.8	concentrated
Mauritius[i]	32.6	16.9		47.5	2.5	1.7	generalized, low level
Mozambique	38.4	10.5	50.4	<0.5	<0.5	12.5	generalized, high level
Namibia	92.3		6.0	<0.5		15.3	generalized, high level
Niger	0.6	90.7	8.7		<0.5	0.8	concentrated

Nigeria	45.9	43.9	9.8		<0.5	3.1	generalized, low level
Rwanda	82.7	7.9	9.0	<0.5		2.8	generalized, low level
Sao Tome & Principe	95.8	3	1.2	2.0	1.0	no data	
Senegal	5.5	87.6	6.2		<0.5	1.0	generalized, low level
Seychelles	96.9	0.1		1.0	1.9	no data	
Sierra Leone	11.5	45.9	10.4	<0.5	2.0	1.7	generalized, low level
Somalia	1.4	98.3	0.1		0.1	0.5	concentrated
South Africa	83.1	2.4	8.4	<4.0	2.4	18.1	generalized, high level
Sudan	16.7	70.3	11.9		1.0	1.6	generalized, low level
Swaziland	86.9	0.7	10.7	1.0	1.2	26.1	generalized, high level
Tanzania	50.4	31.8	16.1	1.5	<0.5	6.2	generalized, low level
Togo	42.6	18.9	37.7	<1.0	<5.0	3.3	generalized, low level
Uganda	88.7	5.2	4.4	1.0	<0.5	5.4	generalized, low level
Zambia	82.4	1.1	14.3	2.0	1.0	15.2	generalized, high level
Zimbabwe	67.5	0.7	30.1	<0.5	1.0	25.3	generalized, high level

Countries in boldface type are majority Christian.

Source: Compiled by author from UNAIDS 2006, 505; UNAIDS 2008b, 215; Barrett, Kurian, and Johnson 2001.

---

[a] Other terms for ethno-religionists are animists or traditional religionists.
[b] This category includes Hindu, Bahia, Buddhist, Chinese Folk Religionists, Coptic Christians, and Jews.
[c] This category includes atheists.
[d] HIV prevalence is the percentage of people between fifteen and forty-nine years old estimated to be HIV positive.
[e] In its 2008 report, UNAIDS provides no data for prevalence rates for Cape Verde, Democratic Republic of Congo, Sao Tome and Principe, Seychelles, and Sudan. For the sake of calculations, I used the data from the 2006 report for the Democratic Republic of Congo and Sudan. There was no data in the 2006 report for the other three countries.
[f] The 2008 UNAIDS report did not include data for the Democratic Republic of Congo or for Sudan. The values in this chart for these two countries are from the 2006 report.
[g] For Kenya UNAIDS only reports data in a range, not a particular estimate. I use the median value when I figure the mean HIV prevalence level for countries classified by religious majority.
[h] There is debate about whether Madagascar has a low-level or concentrated epidemic, because of differences in HIV prevalence data for key population groups.
[i] Mauritius has a unique religious dynamic, with 44 percent of its population being Hindu; 2 percent Bahia; and 1.3 percent Chinese folk religionist.

Table 1.2 Percentage of Countries in Each Epidemic Type, by Religious Majority

Epidemic Type	Countries with Christian Majority	Countries with Muslim Majority	Countries with Ethno-religionist Majority	Countries Without a Religious Majority
No HIV Data (N=3)	11.6	0	0	0
Low-Level Epidemic (N=0)	0	0	0	0
Concentrated Epidemic (N=6)	0	45.4	0	11.1
Generalized Low-Level Epidemic (N=30)	57.6	54.5	50	88.9
Generalized High-Level Epidemic (N=9)	30.7	0	50	0
Total	100 (N=26)	100 (N=11)	100 (N=2)	100 (N=9)

Source: Calculated by author from data from Barrett, Kurian, and Johnson 2001 and UNAIDS 2006, 2008b.

Additionally, wives and girlfriends left without a male breadwinner may have sex with multiple partners to ensure access to food, shelter, protection, or income (*Economist*, June 30, 2007, 91).

One cultural explanation for the Christian-Muslim difference focuses on the fact that some ethnic groups that are predominantly Christian do not practice male circumcision while almost all African Muslims do. Over forty-five observational and biological studies have demonstrated that male circumcision reduces the risk of heterosexual HIV infection. Random controlled trials in Kenya and South Africa were stopped early for ethical reasons because initial findings showed a 60 percent decline in HIV risk for circumcised men (Potts et al. 2008; *Globe and Mail*, March 27, 2008; *Chicago Tribune*, April 23, 2006).[9]

Another cultural explanation highlights the perceived differences in sexual behavior between Christians and Muslims. Here research is less conclusive than the scientific trials on circumcision's benefits. Isaac Addai (2000) demonstrates that in Ghana, Muslim women are less likely to have premarital sex than Christian women. However, this pattern may result because Muslim women marry at a younger age and live in rural areas. Brendan Carmody (2003) reports that even though young Zambian Christians claim that they do not approve of premarital sex, they often engage in it. On the other hand, Peter Gray (2004) finds that Muslim prohibitions about sexual behavior do have a great impact on the average Muslim. Despite limited evidence, both Muslim and Christian leaders have expressed the perception that Muslim communities can control youth sexual behavior (Becker 2007), with the result being a lower HIV rate in Muslim societies.[10]

AIDS is an issue that shapes society, the church, and economies. The data presented show that countries with large Christian populations have been particularly affected by the epidemic. This fact makes it essential for scholars, public health officials, and donors to better understand church responses to AIDS. These responses become even more crucial in light of the rapid increase in the number of Christians in Africa.

The Explosive Growth of African Christianity

While Western Europe and North America have experienced declines or only marginal increases in the number of Christians in the last century, sub-Saharan Africa has witnessed substantial growth. In 1900, there were 8.7 million African Christians; by mid-2005, that number was 389 million, and it is predicted to be over 595 million by 2025. In 2000, 42.7 percent of the sub-Saharan African population was Christian; by 2025, the percentage is expected to be 48.8 (Barrett and Johnson 2001b, 429). Table 1.3 gives the percentage of a country's population that was Christian in 2000, the percentage projected to be Christian in 2025, and the percentage change in Christian population between 2000 and 2025.[11] The table shows that the percentage of Christian believers is expected to increase in thirty-seven countries, to decline in another ten, and to remain the same in one. The average growth rate is 2.2 percent.

Table 1.3 Estimated Change in Christian Percentage 2000-2025, by Country

Country	Percentage Christian 2000	Percentage Christian 2025	Percentage Growth/Decline (2000-2025)
Angola	94.1	97.4	3.3
Benin	28.5	34.7	6.2
Botswana	59.9	66.4	3.7
Burundi	91.7	93.8	2.1
Cameroon	54.2	60.6	6.4
Cape Verde	95.1	99.9	4.8
Central African Republic	67.8	71.3	3.5
Chad	22.8	22.7	-0.1
Comoros	1.2	1.5	0.3
Congo-Brazzaville	91.2	90.7	-0.5
Côte d'Ivoire	31.8	34.6	2.8
Democratic Republic of Congo	95.4	96.3	0.9
Djibouti	4.5	4.1	-0.4
Equatorial Guinea	88.4	89.2	0.8
Eritrea	50.4	50.9	0.5
Ethiopia	57.7	59.4	1.7
Gabon	90.6	89.6	-1.0
Gambia	3.9	3.8	-0.1

(continued)

Ghana	55.4	59.9	4.5
Guinea	4.0	4.6	0.6
Guinea Bissau	13.2	15.2	2.0
Kenya	79.3	82	2.7
Lesotho	91.0	94.2	3.2
Liberia	39.3	43	3.7
Madagascar	49.5	51.8	2.3
Malawi	76.8	79	2.2
Mali	2.0	2.2	0.2
Mauritania	0.3	0.2	-0.1
Mauritius	32.6	35.6	3.0
Mozambique	38.4	42.5	4.1
Namibia	92.3	90.8	-1.5
Niger	0.6	0.6	0.0
Nigeria	45.9	47	1.1
Rwanda	82.7	86.8	4.1
Sao Tome & Principe	95.8	94.7	-1.1
Senegal	5.5	6.2	0.7
Seychelles	96.9	95.9	-1.0
Sierra Leone	11.5	13.2	1.7
Somalia	1.4	0.7	-0.7
South Africa	83.1	83.2	0.1
Sudan	16.7	18.4	1.7
Swaziland	86.9	89.2	2.3
Tanzania	50.4	56.1	5.7
Togo	42.6	48.9	6.3
Uganda	88.7	92.0	3.3
Zambia	82.4	87.8	5.4
Zimbabwe	67.5	73.9	6.4
Average Percentage Change			**2.2**

Countries in boldface were majority Christian in 2000.

Source: Calculated by author from data from Barrett, Kurian, and Johnson 2001

Africa's population growth explains much of this increase (Jenkins 2007, 105). Some countries with the highest predicted growth rates in Christians such as Benin, Mozambique, Rwanda, Tanzania, Uganda, and Zambia have high fertility rates (when defined as the average number of births per woman).[12] By 2025, Nigeria, Ethiopia, Democratic Republic of Congo, Sudan, and Uganda will be among the top twenty-five most populous countries in the world. Nigeria will have over 200 million inhabitants, and Ethiopia, over 100 million (Jenkins 2007, 99).

Yet, demographic change does not provide the full explanation for the increases found in Table 1.3 (Jenkins 2007, 85). The rise of religiosity is a historic theme in Africa. Economic downturns, political uncertainty, colonial repression, and disease have contributed to religious movements, such as Alice Lenshina's *Lumpa* movement during Zambia's period of decolonization or the rise of Nigeria's *Aladura* healing churches during the devastating 1918 influenza epidemic (Becker and Geissler 2007; Gifford 1998, 32; Jenkins 2007, 60). In one sense, the increase in Christianity can be situated in the current context of a weak African state which cannot provide adequate services to its citizens. With Africa becoming increasingly urban, churches may be the only institutions that reach out to those living in squatter communities. In the Kibera slum of Nairobi, for example, there are over three hundred churches for the 600,000 inhabitants that live in an area the size of New York City's Central Park (Bodewes 2009). As Philip Jenkins (2007, 90) writes, "To be a member of an active Christian church today might well bring more tangible benefits than being a citizen of Nigeria."

It is more than just the fact that churches provide believers with services or establish themselves in unfriendly environments. Through their activities and biblical messages, churches provide an alternative vision that contrasts with modernization and capitalism, forces viewed as isolating, violent, amoral, and demonic. Churches strive to build a new and different community (Dilger 2007). The message that an all powerful God controls the world appeals to many Africans who daily face poverty, disease, and death (Gifford 2004). Moreover, some of the independent churches that emerged in the post-colonial era have played a crucial role in shaping the lives of youth and women, two groups in society negatively affected by capitalism (Jenkins 2007, 88, 150; Sackey 2006).

Christian belief is also situated within a larger African worldview that does not separate the spiritual and temporal worlds. This perspective means many Africans see failed governance and poor economies as "signs" that Satan is working to destroy God's world. Christianity is a means to deliver the continent from these forces (Gifford 2004; Jenkins

2007, 145). The language of spirituality is an idiom that resonates with African society's focus on healing, holistic well being, prophecy, and ancestor veneration (Ellis and ter Haar 1998). African Christians pray to a God of power, one who can bring concrete changes to their lives and who combats evil spirits in their present world and in the next (Bornstein 2005). In contrast, Western Christians often emphasize God's compassion and forgiveness.[13] Spirituality is an issue that has divided African and Western churches since the arrival of the European missionaries, with Europeans (guided by rationality) perceiving a constant struggle with the evils of fatalism, superstition, and witchcraft (Jenkins 2007, 143). For Africans, however, the spiritual realm cannot be denied as a crucial component of one's Christian faith.

African Christianity is extremely heterogeneous. Classification schemes can be somewhat tedious, and some scholars have rejected them because of their limited explanatory power (Sackey 2006, 27; Jenkins 2007, 100-105; Kalu 2008, 75). In this book, I refer to some of the major categories of churches, although I do not explain differences in church responses to AIDS merely in light of this categorization. Because readers may lack an overall familiarity with the basic types of African Christian churches, Table 1.4 provides broad categories using the work of Paul Gifford (2004, 20). Christians comprise a majority of the population for countries in bold type. Using data from the *World Christian Trends* and the *World Christian Encyclopedia*, the most authoritative sources on global Christianity, the table provides very rough estimates for the number of adherents in six major categories. The first, Orthodox, includes the ancient Ethiopian Orthodox Church and various Orthodox churches brought by African Americans, North Africans, and Greeks to southern Africa. Orthodox believers are situated in the Horn of Africa, with their largest populations in Eritrea and Ethiopia.

Table 1.4 Estimated Number of Christians in Major Church Categories, by Country

Country	Total Population	Orthodox	Catholics	Old Mission Protestants (Mainlines)	New Mission Protestants (Faith-Mission & Pentecostals)	Old Independents (African Indigenous)	New Independents (Neo-Pentecostals & Charismatics)
Angola	12.9 m	0	9	2 m	414,000	320,000	846,000
Benin	6.1 m	0	1.3 m	230,000	84,000	57,000	153,000
***Botswana**	2.2 m	120	60,000	79,000	29,000	224,000	479,000
Burkina Faso	12 m	0	1.1 m	799,000	635,000	29,000	56,000
Burundi	6.7 m	1,400	3.82 m	800,000	497,000	20,000	19,500
Cameroon	15 mil	1,200	4 m	3.1 m	99,000	257,000	326,000
Cape Verde	427,000	0	417,000	15,000	499	0	13,600
Central African Republic	3.6 m	0	664,000	521,000	0	140,000	257,000
Chad	7.6 m	0	502,000	782,000	17,000	0	82,000
Comoros	593,000	0	5,700	900	0	0	362
Congo-Brazzaville	2.9 m	400	1.45 m	500,000	53,000	190,000	339,000
*Côte d'Ivoire	14.7 m	20,000	2.18 m	760,000	216,000	580,000	807,000
***Democratic Republic of Congo**	51.6 m	8,100	26.3 m	10.6 m	78,000	7.5m	14.9 m
Djibouti	637,000	19,000	8,800	240	0	0	16
Equatorial Guinea	452,000	0	391,000	15,000	3,300	4,000	11,100
Eritrea	3.85 m	1.77 m	130,000	22,000	0	0	3,300
Ethiopia	62.5 m	22.8 m	450,000	8.5 m	1 m	320,000	741,000
Gabon	1.22 m	0	745,000	233,000	12,000	150,000	35,600
*Gambia	1.3 m	450	31,000	6,400	197	2,000	9,100
Ghana	20.2 m	1,600	1.9 m	3.8 m	858,000	630,000	2.73 m
Guinea	7.4 m	0	117,000	70,000	8,000	10,000	41,900
*Guinea Bissau	1.2 m	0	141,000	9,800	347	0	29,100
Kenya	30 m	740,000	7 m	9.4 m	2 m	6m	4.5 m
Lesotho	2.1 m	0	806,000	381,000	25,000	180,000	248,000
Liberia	3.1 m	0	150,000	464,000	152,000	200,000	318,000
Madagascar	15.9 m	4,400	3.6 m	4.33 m	15,000	65,000	251,000
Malawi	10.9 m	4,400	2.7 m	2.37 m	130,000	2m	1.46 m
Mali	11.2 m	0	125,000	82,000	1,600	2,000	15,000
*Mauritania	2.67 m	0	4,000	600	0	1,000	1,900

Mauritius	1.15 m	0	310,000	115,000	112,000	0	3,000
Mozambique	19.7 m	0	3.1 m	1.89 m	684,000	780,000	1.4 m
Namibia	1.72 m	0	306,000	851,000	23,000	120,000	119,000
*Niger	10.7 m	0	19,000	13,000	526	4,000	24,000
Nigeria	111.5 m	3,100	13.4 m	34 m	3 m	6 m	23 m
Rwanda	7.73 m	2,000	3.9 m	2.2 m	636,000	5,000	97,000
***Sao Tome & Principe**	147,000	0	110,000	5,400	3,900	0	14,000
*Senegal	9.5 m	0	440,000	9,900	3,200	500	13,000
Seychelles	77,400	0	70,000	7,100	790	0	50
Sierra Leone	4.85 m	610	169,000	196,000	25,000	36,000	151,000
*Somalia	7.26 m	91,000	200	1,100	0	0	6,800
***South Africa**	40.3 m	150,000	3.35 m	15.1 m	1.77 m	13m	17 m
Sudan	29.5 m	160,000	3.1 m	3.1 m	7,200	70,000	130,000
***Swaziland**	1 m	0	54,000	193,000	53,000	300,000	455,000
Tanzania	33.5 m	12,500	8.2 m	8.1 m	1.4 m	700,000	630,000
Togo	4.6 m	0	1.1 m	480,000	87,000	18,000	110,000
Uganda	21.8 m	32,000	9.1 m	9.2 m	371,000	150,000	760,000
Zambia	9.1 m	6,400	3 m	2.92 m	311,000	215,000	1.3 m
***Zimbabwe**	11.7 m	6,000	1.1 m	1.72 m	164,000	3 m	4.5 m

m= million
Countries in boldface are majority Christian.
Countries with an asterisk (*) have more neo-Pentecostal and charismatic Protestants than mainline Protestants.

Source: Barrett, Kurian, and Johnson 2001; Barrett and Johnson 2001b, 412-413, 428-429.

The second and third categories—Catholics and the Old Mission Protestants, or the mainline Protestant denominations, such as Anglicans, Methodists, and Presbyterians—were introduced by European colonists.[14] Although Africans had already been exposed to Christianity in places like Ethiopia before the scramble for Africa, the European effort was the first widespread attempt to evangelize the continent. Missionaries established health clinics, hospitals, and schools alongside their churches, and they educated many of Africa's first post-colonial leaders. In a classification schema, Catholics are relatively easy to delineate, because of the church's clear hierarchical structure and its links to papal policies. Catholics comprise a sizeable share of the Christian population in Uganda, Kenya, Angola, Mozambique, and Nigeria.

Most mainline Protestants are organized at the country level in denominations; each congregation may make specific decisions about personnel, worship, and programs, but denominations often set broader policies on issues such as pastor ordination. Many mainlines have retained ties to the church in the former colonial country through global institutions, such as the World Lutheran Federation, the Anglican Communion, or the World Communion of Reformed Churches.[15] However, recent disputes between the more conservative African wings and more liberal Western branches within the same church communion, particularly over gender\and sexual orientation, threaten these global ties. For example, in 2005, the Anglican Church in Nigeria broke ties with the Church in Canterbury, the head of the Anglican denomination worldwide, over the issue of ordaining homosexual clergy (Jenkins 2007, 238). Chapter 5 illustrates that these ideological divisions have the potential to create new coalitions between African and Western churches on certain issues, including AIDS.

The fourth category, the New Mission Protestants, includes older Pentecostal churches and the Wesleyan holiness and Calvinist-leaning, conservative churches. Both of these church types have some ties to the West. The Pentecostals were introduced by North American churches that emerged after the Azusa Street Revival in Los Angeles in 1906. Every Pentecostal church emphasizes that God works actively in all areas of life through the Holy Spirit. Pentecostal worship stresses gifts of the Holy Spirit, such as speaking in tongues (glossolalia), healing, and prophesy. Socioeconomically, African Pentecostals differ from Pentecostals in the West and Latin America, regions where they tend to have lower income and educational levels than other Christians. Instead, African Pentecostals are representative of all economic and educational levels (Pew Forum 2006). Examples of the older, established Pentecostal

Churches include the Assemblies of God, the Church of Christ, and the Apostolic Faith Mission.[16]

More conservative churches without the spirit-emphasis of the Pentecostals came to Africa at roughly the same time. Often calling themselves "faith" missions, many were not closely tied to Western denominations. They stressed morality and disciplined living, and they often read the Bible literally. They tended to distance themselves from the problems of the world, and often viewed African cultures and languages as hindrances to spreading God's word. Examples include the Sudan Interior Mission in West Africa, a US-Canadian non-denominational mission, and the Baptists in the Yoruba lands of Nigeria, which had roots in the Southern Baptists of the United States.[17] Their goal was to spread the Gospel, and they often shunned engagement in health and education efforts, unless the programs helped to win converts (Cooper 2006).

The fifth group is the Old Independents, a collection of churches that were either break-off organizations from Western mission churches or independently established, usually by a dynamic prophet. Examples include the Church of the Lord (*Aladura*) in Nigeria, the *Kimbanguists* in Congo, and the many Zionist churches found throughout southern Africa.[18] Part of the problem with fitting these groups into a typology is that some of the other churches question whether these movements are truly Christian. For example, the World Council of Churches debated for years before allowing the *Kimbanguists* into the organization, because the church's founder Simon Kimbangu claimed to be divine. These spirit-filled movements had no links to the Azusa Street Pentecostal experience, making it impossible to state that Pentecostalism or holiness churches came to Africa only from the West (Kalu 2008, 14). Unlike the mission-introduced churches which were perceived as instruments of colonial authority, these churches' independence made them attractive to Africans. They allowed Africans to hold positions of power as pastors, teachers, elders, and deacons, and they sought to blend the Gospel with African cultures and traditional religious practices such as healing, ancestor worship, and acceptance of polygamy, activities which the mission churches shunned (Sackey 2006; Phiri 2001, 23). Their worship incorporated drums and movement, linking it more closely to traditional African religious ceremonies (Omenyo 2008). Over time, many of these indigenous revival groups developed links to classical Pentecostal organizations, had members who founded new spirit-filled churches, and in some countries, experienced state repression. Some, though, have kept a unique emphasis in one part of their ministry, such as spiritual healing or cleansing believers from witchcraft curses. In contrast to the final group in Table 1.4 (the New Independents), they have tended to remain more tied to rural, traditional ways.

The New Independents, comprised of neo-Pentecostals and charismatic churches, are urban based and have not shunned modernity. They utilize technology, engage in consumerism, and embrace the opportunities of the marketplace. Because segregating the neo-Pentecostals and charismatics is difficult, I focus on the neo-Pentecostals.[19] As the fastest growing sub-set of Protestants, they will have nearly 115 million more members in sub-Saharan Africa than the mainline Protestants by 2025 (Barrett and Johnson 2001a, 29). While it is increasingly difficult to delineate these new Pentecostal churches from their earlier counterparts, these new churches exhibit four common traits. First, their charismatic pastors are adept at using media; many of them have TV and/or radio shows. Second, the churches emphasize their international reach, with many establishing branches in other countries. They have located Western partners to sponsor their schools and socioeconomic projects, and they have created international fellowships such as the Full Gospel Men's Fellowship. Third, some of these churches have become massive organizations that include more than Sunday services; as they have branched out into education and service provision, they have required greater church hierarchy (Kalu 2008, 18-19). These mega-churches also provide jobs for members, through building projects and church plantings (Omenyo 2008).

The fourth trait is that many (though not all) preach "prosperity gospel," which stresses that "Christianity entails success" and that "believers have the right to the blessings of health and wealth won by Christ" (Gifford 2004, 48). These messages appeal to predominantly urban populations, who have felt the daily strain of urban problems such as crime and overcrowding, unemployment, and limited state provision of such basic services as water and sanitation. In tough urban environments, poor and middle class African Christians look to God's power to deal with the material challenges that accompany globalization, migration, and capitalism. Although it was partly replaced in the 1990s by a Pentecostal focus on holiness and increased evangelism, prosperity gospel remains an important theme found in newer Pentecostal churches and more broadly, among African Christians (Pew Forum 2010).

In reality, the categories outlined in Table 1.4 do not capture the complexity of African Christianity. Churches change, adapting to new environments and adopting some of their competitors' worship elements and programs. Africa's religious scene experiences continuous hybridization (Meyer 2004, 452; Omenyo 2008; Sackey 2006). Neo-

Pentecostals have led the mission churches to incorporate media, music, drumming, and lively preaching into worship, and they have caused an estimated forty million mainline and Catholic Africans to identify themselves as "charismatic" within their own church traditions (Pew Forum 2006). But the most obvious effect is that the urban-based neo-Pentecostal and charismatic churches have drawn members from both the old and new mission-introduced Protestant churches (Hendricks and Erasmus 2001, 54). Table 1.4 shows that in the thirteen countries with an asterisk, neo-Pentecostals and charismatics outnumber mainline Protestants. Only six of the thirteen countries are majority Christian. The New Independents are making inroads where there had not been a strong Christian tradition, although in some places (e.g., Mauritania and Niger), these populations remain quite small.

Catholics and the mainline Protestants have influenced the New Mission Protestants and the New Independent churches in the areas of service provision and church formal hierarchy. Mainline Protestant and Catholic churches have a long history of social service delivery, partly rooted in their theologies and partly situated in the pragmatic need to attract members when they first came to Africa (Cooper 2006). In contrast, Pentecostals were often viewed as "other worldly," too concerned with the spirit world to devote energy or resources to problems in their current environment. In roughly the last decade, it has become more difficult to delineate Catholic and mainline Protestant churches from new and older Pentecostal churches in terms of their social outreach efforts. For example, the Full Gospel Bible Fellowship Church in Tanzania provides a ministry program to those with HIV/AIDS (Dilger 2007, 59), while Ghana's Church of the Pentecost has set up schools and a university (Omenyo 2008). These "progressive Pentecostals" have reached beyond their own congregants into the community; in doing so, they have accessed global resources and built ties to state officials (Miller and Yamamori 2007). In terms of church formality, some Pentecostal churches also have copied the hierarchical organization of the Catholics and Old Mission churches, and taken on the use of vestments and titles for church leaders (Kalu 2008).

Before leaving this section, I must devote some attention to the terms evangelical and fundamentalist. Paul Freston (2001, 2) uses four criteria to define evangelicals, who can be from any denomination: (1) conversion—emphasis on the need for change of life or being "born again"; (2) activism—evangelism and missionary efforts; (3) Biblicism—the centrality of Scriptures; and (4) crucicentrism—emphasis on the central role of Christ's sacrifice on the cross. Most social scientists define evangelicals as those individuals who self-identify as such (Emerson and Smith 2000, 3). Based on these criteria, many African Christians could be considered evangelical, although some scholars debate the inclusion of the Old Independent churches, such as some Zionists, in this category (Ranger 2008, 5). Use of the term evangelical is complicated by its close link to American politics. As a relatively distinct segment of American society, evangelicals have tended to take politically conservative positions on abortion and homosexuality and have often voted for Republican candidates (Guth et al. 2001; Paul B. Henry Institute 2009).[20] Yet, since most African Christians are socially conservative, this politically oriented definition of the term is not helpful. Because of the word's limited usefulness in the study of African churches and because of its links to American politics, I use the word in two limited contexts: (1) to refer to American churches that have explicitly sought to spread the Gospel in Africa after independence and more recently, have tried to influence donor AIDS programs; and (2) to cite other scholars' use of the word.

The term fundamentalist has been used to refer to individuals of almost any religion (e.g., fundamentalist Muslim, fundamentalist Jew). Historically, Christian fundamentalism was a movement in American Protestantism during the early twentieth century that reacted to secularism, scientific teachings on evolution, and perceived liberal influences in basic Christian doctrines (Wheaton College 2008). More broadly, Christian fundamentalists believe that the Bible is inerrant. Yet, Paul Gifford (1998, 42) writes that "almost all African Christianity is fundamentalist," since most African Christians approach the Bible rather uncritically. Because Africans rarely utilize the term and because it is often used pejoratively to indicate religious people who lack education or discernment, I avoid the word (see Ellis and ter Haar 1998, 182).

Churches as Civil Society Actors… And More

Many students of African politics and society have examined churches through the lens of the civil society paradigm. Rooted in pluralist understandings of politics, this paradigm gained prominence in the 1980s as donors and scholars looked beyond the often corrupt and inefficient African state for agents of political change and socioeconomic development (Gifford 1998, 19; Bratton 1989; Harbeson, Rothchild, and Chazan 1994, 9). Pluralists view the state to be an arena devoid of interests in which organizations compete to achieve benefits; politics is a zero-sum game, with different groups winning at different times. Pluralists often assume that while groups may differ in resources and power, no group can become too powerful because the association builds cross-cutting ties in society (Gyimah-Boadi 2004, 112; Dahl 1956; Truman 1951).

Alan Fowler (1997, 8) defines civil society as the array of people's organizations, labor unions, guilds, development organizations, women's groups, community-based organizations, and religious associations that are situated between the state and the family. These groups may be formal or informal and they are not established to make profits. Some civil society scholars (Bratton 1989; Gyimah-Boadi 2004, 100-108; Skillen 2004, 21) assert that individuals form autonomous organizations to hold government accountable, to influence policy, to provide needed services to society, to get their members elected (or appointed) to positions of power, and/or to carry out a mission that members support. Civil society advocates assume that such groups understand citizens' concerns and represent their perspective because they are rooted in communities (Harbeson, Rothchild, and Chazan 1994, 22).

Some scholars view churches as simply another type of civil society group, albeit a powerful type (Joseph 1993, 231). Daniel Philpott (2004) details how the Catholic Church spoke out against human rights abuses and poor governance in Malawi in 1992; Tristan Borer (1998, 2, 151) explains that the South African Council of Churches mobilized the global church to challenge apartheid. Churches also supply essential services. It is estimated that religious groups provide between 40 percent and 70 percent of health care in sub-Saharan Africa (Haynes 2007, 172; WHO 2007). Because of their ties to communities, religious organizations are the most trusted organizations in African civil society, with 76 percent of respondents in nineteen countries saying they had confidence in these groups. (This number contrasts with the 44% who trust national governments.) (Gallup News Service 2007)

Yet pluralist understandings of churches as civil society actors do not fully illuminate the churches' role in African politics for three reasons. First, because pluralism asserts that the state has no class, racial, religious, or ethnic interests (Kasfir 1998, 7), the paradigm draws a sharp line between the state and civil society. At times, this division may be accurate, as the state attempts to control, co-opt, or repress civil society groups, and civil society publicly confronts the state. Yet, this division does not capture the fluidity between the state and society or between religion and politics (Azarya 1988; Jenkins 2007, 163). Liberia before civil war broke out in 1989 exemplifies the blurred and constantly changing line between religion and politics: political success required membership in a prominent church and "Christianity [became] part of the structures of oppression" (Gifford 1998, 53).

Second, because it is rooted in Western liberalism's focus on autonomy and rationality, the pluralist view that underlies the civil society paradigm does not take into account the norms, beliefs, and values that shape organizations. This is problematic for the study of religion and politics, since "a church's teachings cannot be entirely left aside [in any analysis of churches as political actors since] religion provides definitions, principles of judgment and criteria of perception" (Gifford 1998, 26). A pluralist focus on politics as a zero-sum game may not resonate with religious worldviews that urge believers to strive for peaceful conflict resolution, unity of purpose, and respectful dialogue (Thomas 2005, 212).

Third, pluralism assumes that organizations are bounded entities with members who have a sense of collective identity. The civil society paradigm takes for granted that an already existing collective identity pushes a common agenda for these non-state actors. The paradigm does not investigate the contentious process of group identity formation, yet the tensions embedded in this process affect how (or if) religious groups will mobilize on the issue of AIDS. As Alberto Melucci (1996, 83) writes, "Collective identity, the construction of a 'we', is . . . a strong and preliminary condition for collective action." Because AIDS is tied to questions about morality, relationships, biblical commands, and social justice, the definition of the "we" can be a process influenced by emotion, symbolism, and power inequalities. The pluralist approach to state-church relations may be too static to elucidate this dynamism.

In summary, churches are similar to other civil society organizations in many ways. As one donor official in Zambia pointed out, many of the tasks that churches perform—representing grassroots constituencies, caring for the poor, and challenging the state to be accountable—are things that other civil society groups can do (Interview 13). Yet, church members and leaders view religious organizations as distinct entities that rise above pluralist politics. Throughout my research, interviewees repeatedly asserted that churches have a deep commitment to communities, operate with higher standards, foster hope among the sick and downtrodden, strive for consensus in politics, and do not abandon poor communities in tough times (Interviews 4, 17, 19, 25, 54, 57). While many of these respondents have a biased perspective, their arguments cannot be ignored since they motivate participation in church activities, including AIDS actions. Throughout this work, I consider the ways churches both resemble and differ from other civil society actors in the AIDS fight.

Religion and Development: A New Approach

Since the end of the Cold War, development scholars have paid more attention to religion.[21] To understand this changed perspective, it is important to highlight some elements of modernization theory, the dominant development paradigm from the 1950s until the 1980s. First, modernization theory argued that traditional and religious beliefs would become less important as modern (i.e., Western) education fostered rational decision making in poor countries. Over time, more of the world's people would live in secular environments, and religion, if it existed at all, would be relegated to the private realm (Cox 1968). As the statistics presented earlier demonstrate, this has not occurred and "the world today is as furiously religious as it ever was" (Berger 1999, 3). In fact, because of the global growth of Islam and Christianity, the world is becoming more religious. Atheists and nonreligious individuals were 19 percent of the global population in 1970; by 2025, they are predicted to be 13 percent (Barrett and Johnson 2001b, 4).

Second, modernization theory assumed a secular state would direct a country's development process (Huntington 1968). Yet, state-driven development has not met Africans' expectations; many countries suffer from high debt, dilapidated (or nonexistent) public services, weak governance, and pervasive poverty (Englebert 2009). The rise of military regimes, one-party states, and dictators in many African countries during the 1970s, with the massive corruption and human rights violations that often accompanied these regimes, caused donors to re-evaluate their focus on state institutions as engines of development.

Third, modernization theory touted capitalism, but many Africans believe that the neoliberal structural adjustment policies adopted since the 1980s have had negative consequences. Trade liberalization, privatization, government retrenchment, and cuts in health and education services have contributed to rural-to-urban migration, international migration, unemployment, social pessimism, isolation, and household hardship. They also have not adequately addressed social inequality, poverty, and hunger (Tripp 1997; Manuh 2005, 43; Overa 2007; van de Walle 2001; Moss 2007). While the reasons for these failures are beyond this book's scope (see van de Walle 2001; Stiglitz 2006), it is important to recognize that their failure called into question the inordinate focus on macroeconomic, neoliberal policies that were rooted in the Western development experience (Haynes 2007, 9). The limits of structural adjustment led Africans to look for new alternatives to the state for services, such as religious organizations (Jenkins 2007).

The limits of modernization led many donors to refine their perspectives. By the 1980s, donors had started channeling more funding to civil society organizations, which were perceived to be independent agents of positive political and economic change. Donors realized by the 1990s that faith-based groups, defined to be one component of civil society, had vastly under-utilized potential (Haynes 2007, 7). The difficulty of implementing structural adjustment policies made donors increasingly realize that the development process must engage cultural norms, moral and ethical issues, and local conceptions of political and spiritual power (Thomas 2005, 222). In 1998, the World Bank and the Anglican Church initiated the World Faiths and Development Dialogue, a conference to facilitate cooperation and discussion between donors and faith-based groups. Since then, the Dialogue has established a small organization that has become a voice on normative issues related to program design and service delivery (Marshall 2001; Haynes 2007, 63-64; Thomas 2005, 227-229).

In terms of AIDS, donors have paid more attention to religion since approximately 2001. In that year, all member states of the United Nations signed the Declaration of Commitment on HIV/AIDS at the General Assembly Special Session on HIV/AIDS. The declaration acknowledges that "religious factors" are crucial for HIV prevention and that faith-based organizations provide important leadership in the AIDS fight (United Nations 2001). At the session, faith-based organizations called for greater partnership with governments and international organizations (WCC 2001). Member states reiterated these points at the 2006 follow-up session of the conference.

Building on these actions, UNAIDS co-wrote a report in 2006 with Church World Service, the Ecumenical Advocacy Alliance, Norwegian Church Aid, and the World Conference of Religions for Peace that provides strategies for working with faith-based groups (Church World Service et al. 2006). UNAIDS also hosted a 2008 meeting where various UN agencies and faith-based groups developed a plan for future partnerships. The United Nations invited seventy-three faith-based groups (including forty-one from Africa) to participate in a June 2008 comprehensive review of progress on AIDS.[22] Finally, many 2008 UNAIDS country reports herald the work of faith-based organizations.[23]

Two major global programs that finance AIDS programs—the Global Fund to Fight AIDS, Tuberculosis (TB) and Malaria ("Global Fund") and the US President's Emergency Plan for AIDS Relief (PEPFAR)—demonstrate that donor attention to religion in the AIDS fight has moved beyond rhetoric to include substantial funding and institutions for decision making. Established at the 2001 UN Special

Session on HIV/AIDS, the Global Fund is not a programming entity, but a mechanism for raising and disbursing money. Countries, individuals, and corporations can donate to the Global Fund, which awards grants based on a proposal's technical soundness. Between 2002 and August 2009, the Global Fund had disbursed $8.3 billion to 141 countries in its first seven rounds of funding.[24] Sixty-one percent of these funds had gone for AIDS, 25 percent for malaria, and 14 percent for TB. Sub-Saharan Africa had received 57 percent of the total funds disbursed (Global Fund 2008c).

The biggest funding mechanism for AIDS in Africa is PEPFAR, which provided over $18 billion between 2003 and 2008 for AIDS treatment, care, prevention, and support programs. During its first five years, PEPFAR concentrated its efforts on fifteen countries, twelve of which are in Africa.[25] Its 2003 authorizing legislation required that 55 percent of funding be used for AIDS treatment programs, 20 percent for HIV prevention efforts, 15 percent for care and support, and 10 percent for orphans and vulnerable children. It required that one-third of the HIV prevention money go to programs that teach sexual abstinence and fidelity.[26] In each country, American agencies, national ministries, and the PEPFAR coordinator set annual targets for treatment, care, prevention, and health care capacity building. Some critics initially complained that the Office of the U.S. Global AIDS Coordinator in Washington had a bigger role in setting targets than national governments and that PEPFAR did not consult civil society representatives or other donors working in the focus country. As PEPFAR programs became more established, this particular criticism lessened (Patterson 2006, 144).

In July 2008, the US Congress reauthorized PEPFAR for an additional five years for $48 billion, including $5 billion for malaria and $4 billion for TB. While it retained the 10 percent earmark for spending on orphans and vulnerable children, the reauthorization provided greater flexibility for some of the other targets. In terms of prevention funding, it does not set specific levels for spending on abstinence and fidelity programs, but it does require a country to report to Congress if this spending falls below 50 percent of prevention monies. It requires that at least 50 percent of funding be allocated for treatment and care. It also increases spending to monitor and evaluate programs, and to train 140,000 health care professionals (UCSF 2009).

Unlike the Global Fund, PEPFAR has no formal procedure for incorporating civil society organizations (including faith-based groups) into its decision making. Yet, faith-based organizations have benefited from PEPFAR funding. In 2005, roughly 20 percent of PEPFAR grants went to faith-based organizations (Patterson 2006, 152). This percentage mirrors broader patterns in US foreign aid. In 2006, the *Boston Globe* analyzed 52,000 contracts, grants, and cooperative agreements by the US Agency for International Development (USAID). In 2001, 10.5 percent of USAID dollars went to faith-based organizations; by 2005, this percentage was 19.9.[27] Ninety-eight percent of the USAID money to faith-based organizations has gone to Christian organizations. Most grantees such as World Vision or Catholic Relief Services have years of development experience. Since these international faith-based organizations usually provide sub-grants to African partner churches and community groups, the increased US money to religious organizations has meant African churches have more access to donor funding. Since PEPFAR has pumped millions into AIDS, much of this money for religious groups is slated for programs related to the disease.[28] With the start of the "New Partners Initiative" in 2006, some African faith-based and community organizations also have obtained smaller grants directly from PEPFAR (PEPFAR 2006).

The focus on religion in development has led to greater attention to faith-based organizations in the AIDS fight. As Chapter 4 illustrates, some of these groups have become incorporated into AIDS decision making through Global Fund institutions and national AIDS commissions. Some also have received funding through the Global Fund and PEPFAR. The efforts of UNAIDS, the Global Fund, and PEPFAR are rooted in the growing realization that religious institutions have a role to play in the AIDS fight. Chapter 5 explores the implications of this move for church AIDS activities, church-state relations, and churches themselves.

The Method

This chapter introduced the AIDS issue, highlighting reasons that churches have an interest in the disease and its effects on African societies. It then situated African church actions on AIDS in light of three larger phenomena: the growth in African Christianity; the tendency to view churches as synonymous with other civil society organizations; and increased donor interest in and funding for religious groups in development. The chapter demonstrated that the rise of new churches in Africa and the reform of established ones make the continent's religious landscape fluid. Pluralism tends to ignore the complexity of these religious organizations, and particularly how the secular and sacred realms interact. Greater attention to religion in development has fostered increased involvement of faith-based groups into the AIDS fight, although sometimes this incorporation mirrors pluralist assumptions about religion and politics.

My analysis relies on three sources of data: personal interviews, newspaper articles, and church and donor reports. Between 2005 and 2010, I interviewed over sixty secular and religious AIDS activists, church leaders, donor representatives, and officials with international faith-based organizations in Zambia, Ghana, Kenya, and the United States. Because interviewees were assured of their anonymity, the List of Interviews identifies respondents only by their type of organizational affiliation. These open-ended interviews demonstrate the complexity of church actions on AIDS, and I utilize their insights throughout the book. I also examined African newspaper articles from January 1995 to June 2008 for the twenty-six countries with a Christian majority (see Table 1.1). I conducted a LexisNexis Academic database search using the terms "churches" and "HIV/AIDS." Some countries such as Kenya, Uganda, and South Africa had huge numbers of articles, although not all were relevant. Many stories described the speeches of government and religious leaders, but far fewer described specific church actions on AIDS. This pattern results because news organizations can easily (and cheaply) cover speeches. But it also reflects the nature of African politics, in which individual state and civil society leaders shape political agendas and power centralization heightens the importance of leaders' rhetoric (Hasty 2005, 18, 49; van de Walle 2001). Religious leaders' public pronouncements provide insight into church responses to AIDS. While sometimes confrontational, the speeches are more likely to use praise and persuasion to change public attitudes and policies. These public statements also hint at church activities during private discussions with policymakers.

I acknowledge the limits of using newspapers for data. Not all African newspapers are indexed in LexisNexis, and news sources for Francophone countries are underrepresented. Journalists and editors act as gatekeepers, so not everything churches do or say is covered. The Catholic and mainline Protestant churches are more likely to receive coverage, since their longer histories and well-developed national institutions facilitate ties to news organizations and they often have public relations offices. However, in the age of cheap media technology, more independent media outlets, and the internet, this advantage is disappearing. Leaders of the New Independent Churches are increasingly covered in the news and many have their own websites and online newsletters. Despite these problems, news articles make it possible to discern patterns in church responses to AIDS.

The next chapter begins with a typology of church reactions to AIDS based on timing and scope. I use several cases to illustrate the typology, although I acknowledge that in reality, there is fluidity and dynamism in churches' AIDS actions. Chapters 3, 4, and 5 examine the factors that explain various church reactions to the disease. The book reveals the diversity and complexity not only of church reactions to HIV/AIDS, but also the reasons for those actions.

---

[1] Positive assessments of church involvement on AIDS include Parry 2003; Dilger 2007; Green and Ruark 2008; Global Health Council 2005. Negative assessments include Marshall and Taylor 2006; Fenio 2005; Haddad 2002. Ambivalence about churches in the AIDS fight is evident in Krakauer and Newbery 2007 and Haynes 2007. Several major works on AIDS in Africa by social scientists have ignored churches (see Barnett and Whiteside 2002; Poku and Whiteside 2004; Hunter 2003; Patterson 2006).

[2] See http://www.livinghopeusa.org for more on the Living Hope Community Centre.

[3] Specific biblical references include Luke 18:35-42, Luke 8:43-48, Luke 5:12-15, and Luke 5:17-20.

[4]Specific biblical references include 1Timothy 5:30, Mark 9:36-37, and Luke 18:3.

[5] The countries included in the survey were Côte d'Ivoire, Senegal, Ghana, Ethiopia, Kenya, Uganda, Tanzania, Nigeria, South Africa, and Mali. Respondents were given a list of problems to rank order. Other problems mentioned were crime, illegal drugs, corrupt leaders, immigration, pollution, schools, drinking water, conflict, and emigration (Kaiser Family Foundation and Pew Forum 2007).

[6] Interviewees were assured that they would not be identified in any publications. See the methodology section at the end of the chapter.

[7] Author conversation at the Network for African Congregational Theology Conference on AIDS, Poverty, and the Church in Africa, Lusaka, Zambia, August 4-11, 2007.

[8] For example, Muslims in Ghana and Kenya dispute reports about the size of the Christian population in each country (see US Department of State 2008a).

[9] Circumcision appears to protect against HIV infection in several ways. The foreskin of the penis has a high number of Langerhans cells, a white blood cell which HIV targets; removal of the foreskin removes this entry point for the virus. Additionally, a circumcised penis develops a tough layer of skin that is harder for HIV to penetrate. Circumcised men are less likely to contract other sexually transmitted infections, which increase vulnerability to HIV (*Globe and Mail*, March 27, 2008).

[10] Protestant pastors and seminary professors echoed these ideas about Muslim control at the Network for African Congregational Theology Conference on AIDS, Poverty and the Church in Africa, Lusaka, Zambia, August 4-11, 2007.

[11] The 2025 estimates take into account the number of Christian births and converts minus the number of Christian deaths and defectors.

[12] Birth rates (or the number of births per woman) in 2005 for these countries were Benin (5.9), Mozambique (5.5), Rwanda (5.7) Tanzania (5.0), Uganda (7.1), and Zambia (5.7) (UNDP 2005, 234-235).

[13] This point was repeatedly stressed during a year-long academic reading group on African Christianity composed of African and American faculty at Calvin College, Grand Rapids, Michigan, 2008-2009.

[14] Mainline Protestants are sometimes referred to as orthodox churches. In this volume, I use the term orthodox to refer to the Ethiopian Orthodox Church and orthodox churches in southern Africa.

[15] The organization was formerly termed the World Alliance of Reformed Churches. It merged with the World Ecumenical Council in June 2010 to form the World Communion of Reformed Churches.

[16] Birgit Meyer (2004, 447-450) points out that some of these "established Pentecostals" have sometimes been termed "African Independent Churches," "African Indigenous Churches," or "Africa-Initiated Churches." (All symbolized by the acronym AIC.) To make matters more confusing, some scholars refer to indigenous churches such as the Zionists with the acronym AIC. In order to reduce confusion, I avoid using the acronym AIC. Additionally, the established Pentecostals are sometimes termed "first wave" charismatic churches to distinguish them from Pentecostal movements since the 1980s (see Barrett and Johnson 2001b).

[17] The Sudan Interior Mission is now called Serving in Mission.

[18] For information on these and other African indigenous, spiritualist movements, see Kalu 2008.

[19] These churches are sometimes called Pentecostal-charismatics or third wave Pentecostals.

[20] Some scholars and American evangelicals have asserted that the movement in the West has matured and diversified (Tippett 2008; George et al. 2008).

[21] Religion also has received more attention in the international relations field. Because I frame AIDS as a development issue, however, I focus on the incorporation of religion into the study of development (see Philpott 2004; Huntington 1991, 1996; Thomas 2005).

[22] The seventy-three invitees did not include faith-based groups that already have consultative status with the UN Economic and Social Council. Some denominations (e.g., Presbyterian Church-USA), ecumenical organizations (e.g., the World Council of Churches or the World Evangelical Alliance), and development organizations already had consultative status (for information on nongovernmental organizations at the United Nations, see http://www.un.org/esa/coordination/ngo). Information on invitees is derived from Director, Christian Connections in International Health, email correspondence, April 30, 2008.

[23] For example, reports from Zambia and Lesotho highlight specific actions of faith-based groups (see individual country reports at http://www.unaids.org/en/CountryResponses/Countries/default.asp).

[24] In 2009, the Fund reported that it had approved $18.7 billion in grants. However, because awardees must sign separate grant agreements and meet benchmarks for multi-year grants, disbursed and approved amounts differ (Global Fund 2009).

[25] The twelve African countries are Botswana, South Africa, Namibia, Zambia, Mozambique, Kenya, Tanzania, Rwanda, Ethiopia, Uganda, Nigeria, and Côte d'Ivoire. The 2008 reauthorization kept these focus countries.

[26] According to a health expert involved with PEPFAR in Côte d'Ivoire, even with this requirement, there were some PEPFAR country directors who successfully made the case to Washington that they needed to spend less on abstinence and more on condom distribution. Informal conversation with author, Accra, Ghana, August 20, 2008.

[27] Executive orders issued by President George W. Bush during 2001 made it easier for faith-based groups to apply directly to US agencies for funding (Black, Koopman, and Ryden 2004, 297).

[28] Not all African faith-based groups have been able to access PEPFAR funding, a point of contention among some churches and Muslim organizations.

2
Church Responses to the AIDS Epidemic

During a casual conversation, I told an American missionary working on health care in rural Kenya that my research examined the intersection of African churches, politics, and the AIDS crisis. Throughout our discussion, the individual expressed doubt that I would find much to investigate in my upcoming trips to Zambia and Ghana. The missionary's opinion seemed to be that churches in Africa avoid politics, AIDS, or both.[1] Yet, my fieldwork in those two countries, interviews with leaders of global ecumenical organizations, and an examination of secondary sources of data paint a more complicated picture. Church leaders make public statements about the disease and attend AIDS conferences while congregations organize to mitigate the negative impacts of AIDS and search out donors for funding (Interviews 2, 25). "So much is happening at community and national level[s] in terms of [the] response to HIV and AIDS," said a Catholic aid worker in Nairobi (*Catholic Information Service for Africa*, October 26, 2007). In contrast, one Zambian (Interview 15) bemoaned, "Churches could be doing more," and another said that church responses could be controversial (Interview 16). There tends to be a general consensus that while many religious bodies are doing something about AIDS, more of them still need to become involved.

This chapter outlines a typology of church responses to AIDS, which acknowledges the political nature of these AIDS activities. The typology presented, and the examples of ideal types, challenges the conventional wisdom on church AIDS involvement which asserts that churches provide care, discourage sex, or condemn people with HIV/AIDS (Parry 2003; Pfeiffer 2004; Okaalet 2002; Agadjanian and Sen 2007; Global Health Council 2005). The examples below illustrate that some churches have done more about AIDS than the above interviewees suggest. The typology demonstrates the creative ways that churches mix pragmatic actions such as supporting orphans or lobbying donors for program funding with spiritual activities such as prayer and healing.

These church responses are set within the context of a continuing AIDS crisis in Africa. From the late 1980s through the present, attention to the disease from bilateral and multilateral donors and African states has ebbed and flowed. Successes in the AIDS fight are uneven. Access to AIDS treatment has increased and recipients have benefited from better health and longer lives. Yet, in 2008, an estimated 1.4 million Africans still died of the disease, the same number as in 2001. Infection rates continue to be high. In 2008, 1.9 million Africans were newly infected with HIV, despite increased knowledge about modes of HIV transmission (UNAIDS 2009a). While some countries experienced a decline in prevalence, and while some prevention strategies such as delaying sexual debut and using condoms with commercial sex workers have increased, these changes are not universal. As UNAIDS (2009a, 29) concluded, the "epidemics in the region are much more varied than previously understood." Church responses to the intricacies of the epidemic are nuanced and ultimately, political.

A Broader Understanding of the Political

My conversation with the missionary in Kenya reveals how Westerners often understand politics. While many churches are active on AIDS, their activities do not always resemble the interest group politics of the West. Pluralism assumes that autonomous civil society organizations act in the public realm to influence state decisions (Diamond 1988, 23). Politics is thus viewed as the realm of formal government decision making. Church political activities fit this model when clergy and believers head political parties, hold elected office, and speak out against government policies (Ranger 2008; Borer 1998). For example, Catholic Archbishop Pius Ncube of Zimbabwe condemned the regime of President Robert Mugabe, an action that received national and international attention (*Herald,* July 22, 2004).

On the other hand, African politics often has been characterized by various levels of patronage, power centralization, personal networks, and the hybridization of formal and informal decision-making processes (van de Walle 2001). Politics is extended beyond activities that occur in formal institutions among elected or appointed officials. Because personalities and informal processes matter for politics, church actions and rhetoric which Westerners may consider to be private, local, or apolitical can affect who has access to resources, what values society accepts, how decisions are made, and how individuals become empowered in decision making. Religious leaders may resemble state officials when they use their intangible powers of charisma, moral authority, and personal networks to influence political priorities. While these actions may not directly challenge the state, they are political, since they incorporate power to shape decisions, affect perceptions of state legitimacy, and have the potential to empower citizens. For example, when Reverend Nyansanko Ni-Nku, former president of the All Africa Conference of Churches, called for greater access to AIDS treatment for Africans in 2004, he implied that African states and the international community were not meeting their moral obligations to millions of Africans (*East African Standard*, June 12, 2004). In a less direct, but still political way, when churches help support families of HIV-positive people they may empower those individuals to gain education or other skills for long-term independence. This process may contribute to citizenship development (Miller and Yamamori 2007).

Many African Christians involved in the AIDS fight do not refer to themselves as activists, since the word often has particular connotations that include public challenges to government. Yet, even if they do not use the word activist, religious groups are still involved in processes of trying to bring about a world without new HIV infections and AIDS deaths. The Reverend Canon Gideon Byamugisha (2010), a Ugandan Anglican priest who was the first African religious leader to openly declare his HIV-positive status in 1992, explains that religious groups understand their activism on AIDS to be a "dynamic but coherent process that seeks to achieve socio-cultural, economic, educational, spiritual and political change for a community, nation and world that is safer, healthier, more peaceful, more prosperous and more fulfilling for all God's people."

Church responses to AIDS reflect the fact that political and religious life cannot be easily divided in Africa (Ranger 2008; Gifford 1998). Religion has entered the public square through representation in AIDS policy-making and funding institutions, and through religious leaders such as Reverend Ni-Nku who demand state services or donor attention to AIDS. As politicians from Kwame Nkrumah to Frederick Chiluba recognized, religion is a powerful political asset. Political leaders also have crossed into the religious realm to fight AIDS (Ellis and ter Haar 1998; Ranger 2008). For example, Botswana's Ministry of Agriculture began weekly prayers for those with HIV/AIDS (*African Church Information Service,* November 10, 2003), and the late Zambian president Levy Mwanawasa called on religious authorities to do more to fight the disease (*Times of Zambia*, June 21, 2007). Sometimes the blurring of political-religious lines means that politicians have entered the actual physical space of religion—Sunday morning church services, Friday Muslim prayers, and all-night Pentecostal rallies—to discuss AIDS. In 2007, South African Deputy President Phumzile Mlambo-Ngcuka spoke directly about AIDS to hundreds of jubilant Catholic youth at a mass for National Youth Day (*BuaNews,* January 29, 2007).

A Typology of Church AIDS Activities

To facilitate the analysis of church actions on AIDS, I set up a typology. I recognize the potential pitfalls of typologies: both the danger that readers will interpret categories as static, and the concern that the typology will not capture social phenomenon that fall between the cracks of its categories. Despite these limitations, typologies offer an important analytical tool. They help investigators see patterns and they bring order to issue arenas with multiple actors and activities. This book uses a two-dimensional model, based on the scope and timing of church AIDS activities. In doing so, I acknowledge that not all church actions fit along these dimensions and that churches can change their approach to AIDS over time.

The typology has the advantage of focusing on church actions, which are verifiable and observable phenomena, not normative perceptions of what church activities should be. It also does not rely on an analysis of how churches define the AIDS epidemic. While I agree that "the definition of the [AIDS] problem determines the way [churches] solve the problem" (Paterson 2001, 14-15), I see this "problem definition" (or framing) as only one independent variable that shapes church responses. The next chapter addresses biblical tenets, such as Christian love or God's punishment for sin, that are frames that influence church actions.

I do not classify church AIDS efforts in terms of the level of their intended target, such as a local, national, or global audience. Instead, I recognize that church AIDS actions are dynamic and often multi-faceted; for example, some churches start with congregation-based efforts that expand to include activities at the community or national levels. Other church efforts are national in scope, but have implications for local congregations.

Some readers may expect the typology to classify church AIDS actions based on the substance of those activities—particularly in terms of progressive or conservative positions on controversial issues such as condom distribution, sexual abstinence education, gender empowerment, and/or HIV prevention programs for men who have sex with men. There are six reasons I have not taken this approach. First, there is not enough variation among African churches on these controversial topics for developing a typology because most African Christians are conservative on these issues (Pew Forum 2010). Even church denominations that are perceived to be liberal in the West (i.e., the Anglicans, Presbyterians, and Methodists) have been strongly opposed to condom distribution and strongly supportive of abstinence education. I quickly discovered this point when a Ghanaian church official from one of those denominations lectured me for over fifteen minutes about why "no church in Ghana" would support condoms (Interview 47). The fact that only one church interviewee mentioned homosexuality further illustrates the conservative position of African churches on HIV prevention efforts for this population group. Second, a typology based on church positions on particular AIDS policies could ideologically pigeon-hole churches. For example, most African churches (regardless of the denomination) are conservative on condom distribution, but these "conservative" churches may also provide progressive spaces in which people living with HIV/AIDS can obtain critical care, support, and HIV-related information (Root 2009). Some of these conservative churches have been progressive in their challenges to the AIDS stigma and their openness about how AIDS has affected their congregations and leadership. Thus, it is difficult to label these churches as either conservative or progressive.

A third reason I do not use a typology based on policy substance is that it has the potential to project Western AIDS policy battles onto the African environment. While there are debates on condom distribution or abstinence education in Africa, there are also policy debates over providing state resources for orphan care or deciding who will (or will not) have access to anti-retroviral (ARV) treatment (FBO Roundtable 2009). As one Zambian explained, "The battle over condoms is an American issue, not an issue here" (Interview 11).

Fourth, a typology based on the substance of activities ignores the complexity of church activities, and the often murky line between public proclamations and behind-the-scenes church actions. For example, some churches that have public, anti-condom policies (e.g., the Catholics) have a more nuanced approach in private. Some Catholic AIDS coordinators speak about the necessity of condom distribution, and about their role in referring parishioners to condom-distribution clinics (Interview 41; Catholic Secretariat n.d.; Interview 62). Even many church leaders who exclusively promote abstinence and marital fidelity argue that condoms—and organizations that distribute them—play a role in the AIDS fight (*Zambian Post*, June 16, 2005; April 13, 2002; April 28, 2003; Interviews 1, 2, 7, 9, 10, 13, 14, 32, 41).

Fifth, the typology does not categorize churches based on the substance of particular AIDS activities, because there is often considerable overlap in areas of church actions (see Table 2.1). Prevention and treatment intersect; people must be tested before they can access ARV treatment. With the expansion of ARV treatment and the consequential decline in AIDS deaths in some countries, more home-based care programs are seeking to aid clients with treatment adherence and income-generating activities. And given the large amount of available resources for AIDS in Africa, churches involved in AIDS programs have increasingly become political advocates.

The final reason I adopt the typology based on scope (not substance) of action is because it reflects the empirical evidence from interviewees, who repeatedly focused on the level of church activity on AIDS, not the content of one or two actions. Here it helps to remember that the context for policy debates on AIDS differs from that in the West; African churches are situated in an impoverished environment shaped by neopatrimonial politics, a weak state, and reliance on external donors to fight AIDS. Analysis of the substance of select policies risks ignoring how the socioeconomic arena shapes basic church actions (or inactions). Thus, while the book does not ignore church activities (and differences) on controversial issues such as condom distribution, it asks the broader question of why churches take a narrow or broad approach to addressing AIDS.

While the typology focuses on church actions, I recognize that some churches have done little to address AIDS. They continue to ignore the disease and to deny its presence among church members (Interview 36). They have no activities, and thus, they cannot be classified according to timing or scope. Because this book focuses on church AIDS activities, even if those activities are ineffective, disorganized, controversial, or poorly executed, I spend less time on these "no-action" churches.

The Scope of Church Activities

Church actions may be narrow or broad in scope. AIDS actions are often categorized into prevention, care, support, treatment, stigma reduction, and advocacy, each with a variety of activities (see Figure 2.1). I classify churches that engage in fewer than three of the six categories as having a narrow AIDS focus. Churches with a broad focus engage in three or more categories. I do not assume that churches do all the activities in each category.

Figure 2.1 Types of AIDS Activities

Prevention

- Education on the facts of HIV transmission
- Abstinence education and support groups
- Be faithful campaigns (education and support for fidelity)
- Condom distribution and education
- Education on negotiating safer sex with a condom
- HIV/AIDS education programs in schools
- HIV testing for individuals, groups, and couples
- Counseling (for those infected with and affected by HIV/AIDS)
- Prevention of mother-to-child transmission (through administering nevirapine to HIV-positive pregnant women and providing formula or education on safe breastfeeding)
- AIDS education for pastors and church leaders (formally or informally)

Care

- End-of-life, palliative care
- Home-based care or hospital/clinic-based care
- Assistance with bathing, laundry, food preparation, child care
- Care for orphans through schooling, food preparation, shelter, and psychosocial support

Treatment

- ARV distribution, follow up, adherence education
- Connecting people living with HIV/AIDS to ARV distribution facilities
- Helping people on ARVs adhere to the treatment regimen
- Transportation for people on ARVs to treatment facilities
- Spiritual healing of AIDS (in conjunction with or in lieu of ARV treatment)

Support

- Food, housing, and child care support for people infected with or affected by HIV/AIDS
- Income generating activities for people infected with or affected by HIV/AIDS
- Micro-credit programs for those infected with or affected by HIV/AIDS
- Support groups for people infected with or affected by HIV/AIDS

(continued)

- Prayer for people infected with or affected by HIV/AIDS
- Bible study groups and fellowship for people infected with or affected by HIV/AIDS

Stigma Reduction

- Public statements against the AIDS stigma
- Disclosure by religious leaders of their HIV status
- Support for anti-discrimination efforts such as legislation, discrimination court cases, and legal organizations
- Church policies that discourage discrimination against people infected with or affected by HIV/AIDS

Advocacy

- Representation on government AIDS councils or Global Fund Country Coordinating Mechanisms
- Efforts to link AIDS to structural issues of poverty or gender inequality
- Public demands on national governments to provide more attention or funding to AIDS
- Public demands on donors and/or the international community to provide more attention or funding to AIDS
- Advocacy to governments and donors on issues related to AIDS that are of particular interest to religious groups

---

Prevention includes education on HIV transmission, public awareness campaigns, AIDS education in schools, training for pastors and lay leaders, messages that focus on abstinence or sexual fidelity, and the promotion and distribution of condoms. Prevention programs may urge youth to abstain from sex or to delay their first sexual experience, or they may train women to negotiate condom use with an abusive partner. Many of these programs fall under the broader rubric of behavior change, and they are rooted in the idea that if people have both information about HIV and networks to support changes, they will modify their patterns in sexual relations. The term *behavior change* broadly includes modification in any behavior that increases risk of HIV infection, including multiple sexual partners, sex with a sex worker, intravenous drug use, or sex without a condom with a partner whose HIV status is unknown (Wilson 2006). However, when most church leaders and pastors refer to behavior change, they tend to mean abstinence before marriage and marital fidelity. In fact, many church leaders argue that increased condom use does not fit into a rubric of behavior change, since it facilitates the continuance of multiple sexual relations or pre-marital sex, and it does not require people to modify their actions or commit to relationships (Czerny 2009). On the other hand, since it has been so difficult to encourage condom use in Africa, particularly in long-term relationships, one could argue that increased condom use does constitute behavior change (Epstein 2007; Potts et al. 2008). Because the term behavior change can be understood in many ways, I try to avoid it, unless in direct quotations or when citing interviewees.

Prevention includes testing, which may encompass antenatal testing, routine testing as part of a medical exam, or couples testing before or during marriage.[2] Antenatal testing is a crucial component of prevention of mother-to-child transmission, since HIV can be passed from the mother to the baby during pregnancy, labor, or breastfeeding. If a pregnant woman's HIV status is known, health workers can provide nevirapine to the mother during labor and to the baby after birth to reduce the risk of HIV transmission. HIV-positive mothers can be given formula or be educated about safe breastfeeding.[3]

Care often focuses on home-based care for those with AIDS. For example, the Mtendere Church of Central Africa Presbyterian in Lusaka has a home-based care team composed of both men and women. They are assigned HIV-positive church and community members whom they visit, help with meals and laundry, and connect to other social and medical services (Interview 10).[4] Care also may include providing food, shelter, and/or education for children who have lost one or both parents to AIDS ("AIDS orphans") or other children who are vulnerable to such losses.

Often overlapping with care activities, support is the provision of material, social, psychological, and spiritual help for those infected with and affected by HIV/AIDS. Food supplements or rent payments for families with a breadwinner living with HIV/AIDS are examples. In South Africa, family members who care for AIDS orphans may receive state subsidies (Ewing 2002, 86). In some contexts, support includes income-generating activities or micro-lending to help people with HIV (or their family members) earn money for food or school fees. These impact-mitigation activities acknowledge that some people living with HIV/AIDS face the challenges of poverty, low education, and limited economic opportunities. Churches and secular AIDS organizations have both recognized the need for support groups for HIV-positive individuals (and in some communities, their families); such groups become an arena of comfort, information exchange, and material support. Religious organizations include prayer and biblical reflection in support activities.

Since approximately 2005, treatment with ARVs has become more accessible in Africa. In 1996, scientists discovered that combinations of drugs could stop the ability of the HIV virus to replicate and destroy T-cells, or those cells that fight infection. While ARVs do not cure HIV, they make it possible for people to live longer and be more productive. Because of the drugs' high cost and their patent protection, drug access was limited to the industrialized countries until the success of the treatment access movement (see Smith and Siplon 2006; Halbert and May 2005). The movement was so effective that pharmaceutical companies have lowered their prices, multilateral and bilateral donors have allocated billions of dollars for ARV treatment, and generic production of ARVs has increased greatly. ARV access has become a reality for many HIV-positive Africans. As of December 2007 (the date with most recent figures), 30 percent of HIV-positive Africans who needed treatment had access to it (AVERT 2009). This is a large increase from 2001, when the statistic was only 1 percent. However, this figure masks the fact that some high-prevalence countries actually have widespread access. For example, in Botswana, the number is 79 percent; in Namibia, 55 percent; and in Rwanda, 71 percent (UNAIDS 2009b, 2009c, 2009d).

Some church-based organizations have played a direct role in treatment programs, particularly in countries where mission hospitals provide much of the health care. In those cases, the church-based health care infrastructure distributes ARVs, conducts adherence education programs, and provides continued health assessments of ARV recipients. Even if churches do not provide ARVs directly, they may conduct treatment education efforts and they may use home-based care workers to help clients adhere to the treatment regimen. Because ARVs must be taken with food (and because HIV-positive people live longer with better nutrition), church-sponsored nutritional programs are a crucial component of treatment.

As I describe below, some churches have reacted negatively to treatment because of its focus on scientific healing over spiritual healing. Some church leaders have encouraged those on ARVs to discontinue their use, claiming that true healing only comes from God (Kwansa 2009; Becker 2007). On the other hand, some churches, while suspicious of ARVs, have sought to combine the use of medicines (ARVs) with spiritual healing. HIV-positive individuals may continue to take ARVs, but pastors also use prayer, exorcism, fasting, or traditional herbs to try to drive the virus from the believer's body (Becker and

Geissler 2007, 11). Chapters 3 and 5 further examine this tension between the spiritual and biomedical approaches to treatment.

The high stigma associated with AIDS has led some churches to develop stigma-reduction efforts. Because some of the first individuals to get AIDS globally were homosexuals, intravenous drug users, and sex workers, the disease continues to carry a high stigma (Patterson 2009). Since AIDS has no cure, and since death is often preceded by particularly gruesome physical symptoms (e.g., loss of large amounts of weight, the inability to control bodily functions, and mental delusions), those with the disease have been shunned, ostracized, ignored, or physically harmed (Kelly 2009). While some Christian individuals and churches have perpetuated the stigma, others have sought to reduce it through open discussion, public HIV testing, and disclosure of HIV status (*New Times*, March 17, 2008). Roughly ten years after Canon Gideon Byamugisha disclosed his HIV-positive status in 1992, other African religious leaders formed the African Network of Religious Leaders Living with or Personally Affected by HIV and AIDS (ANERELA+ 2006). In 2006, the organization served as a model for the establishment of the International Network of Religious Leaders Living with or Personally Affected by HIV and AIDS, which serves religious leaders (clergy and lay leaders) in Asia, Europe, and Latin America (Kangale 2009). Because the majority of HIV-positive people are in Africa, ANERELA+ remains separate from the international grouping, although they collaborate closely; between the two, they have over 3,500 members (INERELA+ 2010). The programs of ANERELA+, coupled with some churches' efforts to write AIDS policies for their denominations, provide leadership in addressing stigma. Stigma reduction can also include supporting anti-discrimination efforts, such as legislation on the rights of HIV-positive people to equal treatment in education, housing, or employment (Interviews 16, 20, 21).

Despite such efforts, churches often have not been very successful in stigma reduction; some religious and secular individuals maintain that church AIDS activities contribute to stigma. For example, when churches stress the abstinence and be faithful messages in HIV prevention programs and link these to biblical principles, they imply that those who are HIV-positive have done something immoral. This perspective stigmatizes people living with HIV/AIDS, and may cause them to hide their sero-status and/or to leave the church community (Epstein 2007; Interview 35; Gusman 2009). Support programs may also be built on an underlying suspicion of people living with HIV/AIDS. Several Ghanaian interviewees mentioned that support groups were necessary so that people living with HIV/AIDS would feel acceptance and love, without which they would become angry at society and "willfully transmit" HIV to others (Interviews 29, 35). Such underlying suspicion seemed to advance, rather than challenge, HIV stigma.

More recently faith-based organizations have recognized the need for advocacy to fight AIDS. In the African context, advocacy may be confrontational, but it is usually quite subtle. Often, it is based on personal networks, consensus-building, informal discussions with state actors, or very indirect criticisms of policies. Avenues for such advocacy include media statements about AIDS, church-state meetings about AIDS programs, community meetings, or church representation on decision-making boards that allocate AIDS resources or shape policies. Advocacy can also be aimed at international actors, such as UNAIDS, corporations, or bilateral donors. Churches have tended to be more outspoken and direct in international-level debate than national-level advocacy (*Catholic Information Service for Africa*, October 12, 2007, November 5, 2007; AACC 2008; *National Council of Churches USA News*, October 28, 2003). This pattern may reflect the fact that behind-the-scenes networking is more difficult at the global level, while outward challenges to the state are viewed as too confrontational at the national level. Such advocacy trends may also demonstrate ambivalence among churches and church leaders over the ways that political participation relates to the Christian calling to preach and spread the Gospel. Chapter 4 further addresses these political dynamics.

The Timing of Church Activities

The second criterion of the typology is the time period when the church began its AIDS efforts. Africa's first AIDS cases were recognized in the mid-1980s. Some churches began to act early, particularly in the provision of home-based care and support. Some of these church efforts expanded, while some declined. I use the year 2001 to divide early and late church actions. While the temporal division is somewhat artificial (and some churches in the "late" category had individual-level efforts by pastors or believers before 2001), there are several good reasons to use 2001. In terms of epidemiology, the magnitude of AIDS only became apparent during the late 1990s. By then, the millions of Africans who were infected with HIV during the 1980s had developed AIDS (Iliffe 2006). The increased morbidity and mortality put a huge strain on health services, communities, and families and made it more difficult for churches to ignore AIDS.

AIDS also had become an issue of global and national concern by 2001. Despite early political interest in AIDS in the 1980s, the issue dropped off the global agenda during the 1990s, funding dramatically declined, and most African politicians and religious leaders remained silent about the disease (Patterson and Cieminis 2005; Patterson 2006; *Daily Telegraph*, March 18, 2006).[5] By 2000, changes began to occur. First, the World Bank developed the Multi-Country AIDS Program Initiative (MAP Initiative), which gave countries grants to set up strategic AIDS plans with a multi-sectoral approach and to form national AIDS councils. While the World Bank initiative was criticized for a "cookie cutter" approach to AIDS policy-making and for weakening health ministries (Putzel 2004), the infusion of money and the development of high-level AIDS institutions helped place AIDS on national political agendas. Second, African leaders began to publically discuss AIDS. Encouraged by UN Secretary General Kofi Annan (a Ghanaian) and the new MAP Initiative, African state leaders met in 2001 in Abuja, Nigeria for the African Summit on HIV/AIDS and Other Related Infectious Diseases. At the summit, African leaders promised to "place the fight against HIV/AIDS at the forefront" and "to commit ourselves to take personal responsibility and provide leadership [on AIDS]" (*Africa Recovery*, June 2001). Leaders vowed to involve people living with HIV/AIDS in policy-making and to devote 15 percent of their national budgets to improving health care (Patterson and Cieminis 2005). Third, as mentioned in Chapter 1, the UN General Assembly Special Session on HIV/AIDS produced the Declaration of Commitment on HIV/AIDS that outlined goals for reducing HIV infections and treating people living with HIV/AIDS. All 189 UN member states signed the declaration without reservation, signaling strong support for international action on AIDS.

Fourth, transnational religious organizations also expressed greater concern about AIDS, although the Catholic bishops in southern Africa began to issue communiqués about AIDS as early as 1987 (Czerny and Vitillo 2005-2006). At a 1989 Vatican AIDS conference, Pope John Paul II called for solidarity with individuals suffering from AIDS and for local, national, and international efforts to address the disease (Overberg n.d.). While these Catholic statements seem to have had some effect on church AIDS actions at the national and sub-national levels, early Protestant statements had less impact. During the late 1980s, the World Council of Churches, an ecumenical body formed after World War II and composed of over 350 Protestant churches and denominations in more than one hundred countries, developed statements on AIDS, particularly in response to the AIDS crisis in the West. However, it was only after a 2000 meeting between Medical Assistance Program International, the World Council of Churches, and

UNAIDS that ecumenical action among mainline Protestants increased (Chitando 2007). As Chapter 5 details, the World Council of Churches, as well as the World Evangelical Alliance, developed political advocacy efforts on AIDS and poverty reduction and they sought to educate church members and leaders about the disease. Additionally, evangelical churches in the United States with links to African churches became more interested in AIDS (Patterson 2006; Guth et al. 2001). The national- and global-level efforts raise important questions: Why did some churches address AIDS before 2001, while others acted later?

Figure 2.2 illustrates the typology and provides examples in each category. Because I use these cases throughout the book, I describe them in detail below. While one case is regional in focus, three are church actions situated in the specific countries of Ghana, Zambia, and Uganda. I recognize the limits of focusing on case studies from select countries, and I do not assert that these cases represent all African church activities on AIDS. Yet, the cases from Ghana, Uganda, and Zambia provide enough variation to be broadly representative of different African regions (East, West, and southern Africa) and various AIDS epidemics. As Table 1.1 shows, in 2007 Ghana had an HIV prevalence of 1.9 percent; Uganda, 5.4 percent; and Zambia, 15.2 percent. This diversity permits analysis of the ways that a country's particular epidemic affects church AIDS activities.

Figure 2.2 Typology of Church AIDS Activities

Narrow Focus (<3 activities)	
Pre-2001	Christian Council of Ghana, Compassion Campaign (2000-2003)
Post-2001	Makerere Community Church, Kampala, Uganda (Pastor Martin Ssempa)
	Spiritual Healing Churches
Broad Focus (≥ 3 activities)	
Pre-2001	Catholic Church, southern and eastern Africa (~1987-present)
Post-2001	Northmead Assembly of God, Lusaka, Zambia (Bishop Joshua Banda)

I acknowledge three limits of the case studies. First, none examines church AIDS activities in a country such as Senegal, Niger, or Somalia with a Christian minority and Muslim majority. Because most Muslim countries have relatively low HIV prevalence (see Table 1.1), all religious groups' AIDS activities in those countries have tended to be less pronounced. (Senegal is an exception. See Green 2003) Boubacar Sambo, Michelle Fraser, and Souleymane Issoufou (2008) report that both Muslim and Christian organizations working on AIDS in Niger faced similar challenges because of the country's low HIV prevalence (0.8%), which pushed AIDS off the public agenda. In the Nigerien case, it was impossible to disentangle the effects of low HIV prevalence on church AIDS activities from the effects of religious minority status. To partially address the absence of a Christian-minority country, my cases present some variation in the size of the Christian majority. Ghana has a much smaller Christian majority (55%) than Uganda (88%) or Zambia (82%).

The second limit is the lack of a case of church mobilization from Francophone Africa. There are two reasons for this omission. One of the book's underlying questions is the ways that global Christian movements relate to African church actions on AIDS. However, partly because these post-Cold War movements have been dominated by American faith institutions, many of them have been more active in Anglophone than Francophone countries (Lynch 2010).[6] A second topic of analysis is the relationship between the state and church-run health care facilities. While religiously based facilities exist throughout Africa, they are more prevalent and better resourced in Anglophone countries such as Ghana, Zambia, Kenya, and Uganda (ACHA 2009). To supplement the three country-based case studies, Chapter 4 incorporates cross-national analysis of church actions at the national level.

Third, the case studies do not include every type of Christian church outlined in Chapter 1. The cases examine Catholics, Old Mission Protestants (through analysis of an ecumenical council), New Mission Protestants (through analysis of an Assemblies of God church), and New Independents (through analysis of a neo-Pentecostal church). However, I omit Old Independent Churches, such as the Zionists. I do not want readers to infer that these churches are not active on AIDS. In recent years, some have developed AIDS activities, while others have worked in coalitions with a variety of Protestant churches (Krakauer 2004; Lubaale 2008). But analyzing their efforts is somewhat difficult because these churches are often decentralized and rural-based. Historically, they have shunned participation in public politics, a fact that limits their visibility on AIDS policy-making (Garner 2000a). Because of these challenges, I do not include them.

Case Studies

Churches that Took No Action

Despite the almost three decades of documented AIDS cases in Africa, there are still churches in all the Christian categories that have done little or nothing to fight the disease. Inaction results for several reasons. Many churches are ill equipped to meet the high demands for care, support, treatment, prevention, advocacy, and stigma reduction, particularly in high HIV prevalence countries (Interviews 3, 9, 14, 35, 47, 50, 53; ARHAP 2006). Church members are confused about *how* they should react, and while parishioners may provide an HIV-positive neighbor or friend with support on an ad hoc and individual basis, such activities have not been organized into church programs. Some church members can barely care for their own sick family members or surviving children and widows. They have neither the time nor the energy to combat stigma, to engage in HIV awareness programs, or to lobby the state or donors for better AIDS policies.[7] Interviewees described how the high mortality and morbidity rates in southern African churches have had a negative impact on pastors' health and personal relationships. Many church leaders report problems with sleeping, marital tensions, depression, and increased alcohol use (Interview 9, 10). The pandemic has left some church leaders and members with feelings of hopelessness and impotence.

Other churches have not acted because their members remain uncomfortable with the disease, discussion of its sexual transmission, and exposure to HIV-positive people. Since they often view AIDS as a disease that affects non-Christians or people with little faith (Katongole 2005), they deny its presence in the church. For example, a women's group leader in the South African Nazareth Baptist Church (Shembe Church) explained: "In the Shembe Church, no one has been found with AIDS." Yet, the woman's daughters were sick with TB, a common co-infection of HIV (Krakauer and Newbery 2007, 31). Such churches may sometimes have outreach programs to sick and dying people outside the congregation, perpetuating a view that AIDS is something that "happens to other people" (Paterson 2001, 2).

As more African Christians have become sick with or died from AIDS and people learn more about the disease, silence has replaced explicit denial or the direct shunning of HIV-positive people (Interview 53). The silence pattern means that many pastors do not talk about AIDS, and if congregants are HIV-positive, they quietly hide their status or leave the church. Parishioners may have suspicions about those who are ill, but no one raises the issue of AIDS (Kelly 2007). The lack of public discussion breeds uncertainty for HIV-positive congregants: "You do not know how you will be received if you disclose your HIV status. Will you be accepted? Will you be shunned? Not knowing makes people remain quiet" (Interview 20). For some HIV-positive Christians, the church becomes the last place to which they would turn for help (Paterson 2001; Interview 29).

Churches that Had an Early, Narrow Focus

While AIDS negatively affected Christians throughout Africa, not all churches acted early in organized ways. For those that did, some early efforts peaked and declined, while others blossomed into additional activities. The Compassion Campaign in Ghana provides an example of an early action that included prevention efforts and stigma reduction. The campaign illustrates that while some churches acted early on AIDS, there may be larger contextual, organizational, and political variables that prevent them from expanding their efforts.

In 2000, the Christian Council of Ghana (an ecumenical organization formed in 1929 and composed of fifteen denominational members and two organizations) developed the Compassion Campaign, a four-phase effort independent of the state which incorporated Protestants, Catholics, and Muslims.[8] While the campaign resulted from several factors, the experiences of the Salvation Army and its staff were crucial for the campaign's inception (Interviews 26, 43, 50). By the mid-1990s, the Salvation Army's clinics in central, eastern, and Ashanti regions (areas with the highest HIV prevalence in Ghana) were encountering more patients (particularly women) with AIDS. Clinic staff personally witnessed how AIDS isolated its victims from society and their families. While the clinics provided palliative care, staff quickly realized that "bringing those with AIDS hope in the midst of hopelessness" and "spiritually preparing them for death" were huge components of their jobs (Interview 26). As the clinics grappled with AIDS on the ground, most Ghanaian churches refused to discuss AIDS, believing that people with HIV/AIDS were "dying of sin" (Interviews 27, 29, 30, 35, 43, 45, 49, 50). While AIDS hit some communities hard, in many parts of the country (particularly among middle-class individuals in Accra), there was little, if any, honest discussion about the risk of HIV infection. While "98 percent of Ghanaians knew about HIV," most thought only those who travelled outside the country or engaged in behavior such as prostitution were most at risk (Interviews 26, 35, 39).

To raise awareness, the Salvation Army collaborated with German and Canadian donors to make a docu-drama "Shared Concern" that detailed the plight of HIV-positive Ghanaians. While in 2010 the film seems extremely dramatic (and perhaps a bit discriminatory toward people living with HIV/AIDS), in 1999, it "really shook Ghana" when it was shown on national television and discussed on national radio and TV call-in shows. Callers expressed both fear about AIDS and ignorance about the negative effects of discrimination and stigma on people living with HIV/AIDS (Interview 26).

As a result of the Salvation Army's experiences and the public reaction to the film, the Christian Council of Ghana, the Ghana AIDS Network, and major donors (particularly USAID) met to discuss next steps. One church leader said, "We asked ourselves, 'What could we do as religious institutions that would be a unique approach to AIDS? Something that would be different, versus other NGOs'" (Interview 35). While secular AIDS organizations were working on condom distribution and AIDS education, religious groups had yet to become involved. To address this problem, the campaign first organized a series of workshops for high-level Christian and Muslim religious leaders. One involved individual said, "We knew we'd never get anywhere if we didn't get them to accept that AIDS was real" (Interview 49). The workshops allowed the officials to interact directly with people living with HIV/AIDS: "They soon realized that Sunday school teachers, youth group members, and church women's group presidents all had AIDS" (Interview 30). The campaign's second phase included workshops with 3,000 clergy and lay leaders at the congregational level, so they could build the topic of AIDS into their church activities and messages. The campaign provided manuals, teaching materials, and several training workshops. Church leaders were urged to "discuss [AIDS] anywhere they found themselves" (Interview 35).

The third phase was a public media campaign that urged people to break the silence on AIDS and to show compassion and suspend judgment toward those infected with and affected by HIV/AIDS. Some of the television ads showed religious leaders embracing people living with HIV/AIDS. While there were people who thought the ads were a bit superficial (Interview 50), many said the spots were powerful. One HIV-positive Ghanaian said the campaign's emphasis on "Who are you to judge?" gave him the courage to "come out [about my HIV status] and move forward" (Interview 28). The public campaign was very helpful for Christians who were "wavering" between understanding AIDS as a health issue, which would mean people with the disease needed compassion, and perceiving AIDS as a curse from God (Interview 49).

The campaign's final component was that several denominations, particularly the Presbyterian Church of Ghana and the Evangelical Presbyterian Church of Ghana, wrote AIDS policies, which clearly stated that AIDS is a disease, not a spiritual curse, and which called for compassion, prevention efforts, and nondiscrimination. (The Catholic Secretariat already had such a policy.) In 2005, the Christian Council also issued a detailed policy, which acknowledged the need for confidentiality in HIV testing and counseling and discussed the role of gender inequality in HIV vulnerability (Evangelical Presbyterian Church n.d.; Presbyterian Church of Ghana 2002; Christian Council of Ghana 2005). These statements can be viewed as part of the Christian Council's larger stigma reduction efforts.

There is anecdotal and survey evidence that the Compassion Campaign had some positive effects. Some interviewees (26, 43, 49, 50) agreed that at a minimum, the campaign "made the church wake up" and realize that "AIDS is us" and "AIDS is real." One church leader maintained that now there is less discrimination *within the church* toward those with HIV (Interview 30). A study published in 2008 found that negative attitudes toward people with HIV and AIDS declined between 2001 and 2003, and that this decrease was positively associated with exposure to the Compassion Campaign (Boulay, Tweedie, and Fiagbey 2008). The public role of religious groups in the campaign then thrust them into formal policy-making roles, as the Christian Council, Catholic Secretariat, Pentecostal Council, Council for Independent Churches, and Traditional Healers' Association gained representation on the Ghana AIDS Commission Steering Committee, which makes day-to-day decisions about AIDS (Interview 27). However, it is uncertain whether churches utilize these positions to affect policies. Interviewees, for example, pointed out that churches do not agree with the Commission's comprehensive HIV prevention program, which includes condom distribution and advertisements, yet they have not been able to change the policy (Interviews 38, 47).

When USAID funding for the campaign ended around 2003, the Christian Council started to focus its efforts at the local level on behavior change (abstinence and fidelity) and stigma reduction (Interview 35). Yet, by 2008 when I conducted interviews in Ghana, church efforts seemed minimal and underfunded. Many of the central figures in the Compassion Campaign no longer worked on AIDS; they had moved on to higher education or new policy domains such as malaria prevention and small arms reduction. Some individuals expressed "burn out" with AIDS, while others reported that AIDS is no longer dynamic and urgent, since HIV awareness is high (Interviews 26, 43). Many said that five years after the campaign ended churches were "doing little" on AIDS (Interviews 26, 36, 43, 50). They pointed to gaps in church AIDS efforts, such as the unwillingness to develop (or to adequately fund) care and support programs for people infected with or affected by HIV/AIDS and the continued discomfort with discussions of sex, which is essential for honest and comprehensive prevention efforts (Interviews 29, 30, 36, 52). Others working on AIDS outside of the church complained that while churches were willing to promote compassion in a broad sense to others, they are "unwilling to be proactive" on more specific aspects of the AIDS fight (Interview 34). In the next three chapters I will analyze why Ghanaian churches acted early, but narrowly, and I will suggest reasons why these efforts then declined.

Churches that Had an Early, Broad Focus

As a huge organization with more than 120 million African adherents, the Catholic Church is a substantial actor on the AIDS issue. This is particularly the case in southern and eastern Africa, where countries have high HIV prevalence and sizeable Catholic populations (see Tables 1.1 and 1.4). Catholic programs were some of the earliest and most comprehensive in these regions. Such activities often began with care and support, which emphasized that programs should look after the physical, emotional, spiritual, mental, familial, and community aspects of the person (Rasmussen 2009). Holistic patient care included home-based care, income-generating activities, home visits, spiritual guidance, care for orphans and support for caregivers, food distribution, rent payments, prayer, and distribution of the sacraments (Czerny 2007, 102). While other church-based programs have emphasized a holistic approach to AIDS (and more broadly, socioeconomic development) in the last decade, the Catholic Church was the first to incorporate this comprehensive understanding into AIDS programs (Interview 55; Bornstein 2005).

Efforts in the Ndola diocese of Zambia provide an illustration. In 1991, the diocese began a home-based care program that utilized five hundred volunteer community workers in twenty-five townships. By 2009, the program had over seven hundred volunteers, 95 percent of whom were women (Fikansa 2009). The program integrated palliative care, treatment for opportunistic infections, assistance for orphans and vulnerable children, prevention messages, and spiritual support. By training church and community members, the Catholic home-based care program broke through the African perception that caring was only a family responsibility, and it invested the church in the health of all community members (Iliffe 2006, 105-106). Since the program's inception, the diocese has served over 150,000 people living with HIV/AIDS, and home-based care workers have provided emotional and spiritual support so that many of these individuals could die with dignity (Fikansa 2009). The efforts of this diocese became a model for other Catholic, Protestant, secular, and governmental efforts throughout the region. By 1998, there were eighty-five home-based care projects in Malawi. By 2000, Catholics in Namibia ran southern Africa's largest home-based care program, with thirty-nine staff and over one thousand volunteers (Iliffe 2006, 106-108). The introduction of ARVs has led these programs to increasingly move from palliative care for the dying to psychosocial support for those on ARVs. This transition has brought new challenges since some HIV-positive individuals on ARVs feel healthy and no longer want to participate in programs associated with a stigmatized disease. Instead, these individuals just want to "get on with life" (Fikansa 2009).

Catholic Church involvement in ARV treatment efforts varies between countries. The aforementioned Ndola diocese, for example, does not provide ARVs. Instead, as of 2009, it helped 6,000 people on ARV treatment with nutritional supplements, transport to medical appointments, and treatment adherence; it also conducted counseling and testing at its clinics and referred individuals to government hospitals for ARVs (Fikansa 2009). On the other hand, the Catholic Church in South Africa has become the country's largest ARV treatment provider after the government. Even before the government, PEPFAR, and the Global Fund began to provide ARVs, the Catholic Church collaborated with Médecins sans Frontières (Doctors Without Borders) on treatment projects. These efforts, which showed that ARVs were effective for children and adults and that patients could adhere to a treatment regimen, challenged the South African government to provide free access to ARVs for all citizens who needed them (Joshua 2009).

In terms of prevention, the Catholic position against condom use, even for sero-discordant married couples, is controversial; it has been criticized by both Catholics and non-Catholics. In 2009 Pope Benedict heightened global attention to the condom disagreement when he publicly stated that the AIDS pandemic was "a tragedy that cannot be overcome by money alone, that cannot be overcome through the distribution of condoms, which even aggravates the problem" (*Daily Telegraph*, March 17, 2009). For critics of the Catholic Church's position, such a statement ignored the fact that condom use can save lives through prevention of HIV infection. Critics question how a religious institution which claims to promote the sanctity of life can ignore the complexities of sexual relations, particularly in the African context where poverty and gender inequality may force women to engage in sexual relations to survive and where migration and urbanization have contributed to the decline of social networks that may prevent multiple sexual partners (Epstein 2007; Iliffe 2006; Campbell 2003; *Washington Post*, March 19, 2009). Defenders of the official Catholic position situate the prohibition against condom use in the larger context of church doctrine on contraception, which emerged in 1968 (Supreme Pontiff Paul VI 1968). Church supporters assert that condom use does not urge individuals to develop long-standing, permanent relationships built on trust and love before they engage in sexual relations. For supporters of the church's position, condom use is not "life promoting," since a crucial part of life is the building of trusting relationships. They also assert that the evidence demonstrates that abstinence and marital fidelity are the most reliable ways to prevent HIV infection (Interview 23; *Catholic News Agency*, May 19, 2009; *Washington Post*, March 29, 2009).

While the media sometimes narrows Catholic prevention efforts to include only the church's condom prohibition, the Catholic Church has sought to urge HIV prevention in other ways. Many Catholic health facilities provide voluntary counseling and testing and programs to prevent mother-to-child-transmission. The Catholic prevention of mother-to-child transmission program in South Africa, for example, started in 2001, roughly two years before the government and international donors began to systematically address this means of HIV transmission.[9]

The Catholic Church has tried to reduce stigma in several ways. African bishops have issued over sixty statements on AIDS since 1987. More broadly, through their long-standing involvement on the AIDS issue, the Catholic Church has demonstrated that it is not afraid to tackle AIDS. In most African countries, the Church has internal policies for working with HIV-positive parishioners and employees (Interview 23; *Nation*, June 5, 2000), and it has engaged in deep theological reflection on AIDS. For example, the African Jesuit AIDS Network provides opportunities for Catholic theological networking across the continent in order to facilitate one voice on AIDS.[10]

Overall, the Catholics have been the most active church in terms of political advocacy on AIDS policies (Interviews 5, 55). In South Africa, Catholics publicly challenged the government to provide nevirapine at state-run clinics in order to prevent mother-to-child transmission (Joshua 2009). In Kenya, the Catholic Church called on governments to begin parallel importation of generic versions of ARVs, arguing that the government is morally obligated to request drugs that can help those suffering from HIV/AIDS (*Nation*, May 13, 2001). It also participated in AIDS curriculum development for Kenyan secondary schools (*Nation*, July 22, 2000). In 2005, archbishops and primates from Uganda, Kenya, Tanzania, Rwanda, Burundi, and the Democratic Republic of Congo publicly called for governments to ensure that ARVs were available and affordable to those who need them (*Monitor*, April 7, 2005). On the international level, the Pope has called for compassion, care, nondiscrimination, and acceptance for those with HIV/AIDS (Overberg n.d.). The Catholic Church is credited for being one of the few civil society organizations to react to AIDS after the disease first emerged in Africa (Gill 2006, 128; Epstein 2007). These efforts demonstrate a broad, early AIDS response.

Churches with a Late, Narrow Focus

While some pastors and parishioners in late-acting churches were involved with AIDS before 2001, churches in this category began systematic, formal AIDS efforts after the disease received more national and international attention and after its magnitude had become difficult to ignore. These churches have tended to concentrate on one or two of the components listed in Table 2.1. Churches that focus on spiritual healing as a cure for AIDS are one example of this response. While many Pentecostal churches and/or pastors focus on healing, not all of them claim that they can *cure* AIDS. A minority believe that because evil spirits cause AIDS, prayer camps, hard labor, exorcism ceremonies, fasting, laying hands on the person with HIV/AIDS, and drinking traditional herbs will drive the evil spirits from the believer's body (*Daily Graphic*, September 25, 2008; *New Vision*, September 20, 2006; *Monitor*, July 28, 2007; *Monitor*, October 9, 2007; *East African Standard*, May 25, 2006; *Nation*, May 22, 2006). This focus on healing may lead pastors to urge HIV-positive individuals to quit taking their ARVs (Kwansa 2009; Interview 47; Asamoah-Gyadu 2005b). While healing ceremonies have existed since the first AIDS cases emerged, I categorize this response as relatively recent because it can be viewed as a reaction to the increased use of ARVs. This biomedical solution has made some religious leaders fearful that increased ARV access in Africa will discredit or downplay the spiritual aspects of health and wellness (Kalipeni, Muula, and Liwewe 2009). Spiritual healing also presents a relatively recent challenge to the African state and international donors who support ARV treatment as a major component of AIDS programs. In response, the state and donors have ignored, shamed, repressed, and, in a few cases, sought to understand these churches' healing emphasis (Asamoah-Gyadu 2005b; *New Vision*, August, 29, 2007; *New Vision*, July 10, 2007; *Mmegi/The Reporter*, March 7, 2005).

Not all churches in the late-narrow category have challenged ARV efficacy through spiritual healing. Others have concentrated on prevention or care. The Makerere Community Church in Kampala, Uganda is a church with narrowly focused, recent AIDS efforts that specialize in prevention programs, particularly abstinence and fidelity education. While the church has a few care and support programs for orphans and HIV-positive community members, these are small scale (Gusman 2009). The church was founded by the dynamic Pastor Martin Ssempa in the late 1990s. One of Uganda's neo-Pentecostal churches, its congregation is located near Makerere University and its target audience is primarily university students. In comparison to several other Kampala-area Pentecostal churches, Makerere Community Church is relatively small; average attendance at a Sunday service is roughly three hundred. In his speeches and on his website, Ssempa critiques the "abstinence stigma," or the "negative, biased, hostile attitude … toward those who choose abstinence. . .Abstinence stigma makes young people making healthy choices feel ostracized, embarrassed, isolated, rejected and shamed" (Ssempa 2009). The pastor is a vocal opponent of condom use and became notorious when he publicly burned a box of condoms during freshmen orientation week in September 2004. As the box burned, he reportedly prayed, "I burn these condoms in the name of Jesus" (Epstein 2007, 195, 301-302). He sees condom distribution as a factor contributing to AIDS: "The more we know about condoms, the more HIV we have" (*Monitor*, January 24, 2007). To spread the church's prevention messages, Ssempa hosts a television program (*Monitor*, March 10, 2004). His efforts also have spawned the Campus Alliance to Wipeout AIDS, an organization which has received funds from the US-based Children's AIDS Fund, the Global Fund, and PEPFAR (PEPFAR 2007; *New Vision*, January 13, 2006).

As the central leader of the Makerere Church, Ssempa engages in national and international-level political advocacy on AIDS policies. He has spoken at several evangelical churches in the United States.[11] In 2005, he testified before the US House of Representatives Committee on International Relations on PEPFAR and argued that abstinence had been crucial in bringing down Uganda's HIV rate from 15 percent in 1990 to 5 percent in 2001 (UNAIDS 2009e).[12] In his testimony, he asserted that

Western racism in donor agencies such as UNAIDS and USAID prevents their officials from valuing African solutions to AIDS such as abstinence and marital fidelity (Ssempa 2005). As part of Ugandan First Lady Janet Museveni's Task Force on AIDS, Ssempa has helped to redesign AIDS education programs for schools to place greater emphasis on abstinence before marriage and marital faithfulness (Human Rights Watch 2005). Since 2007, he has become a more vocal opponent of homosexuality.

Ssempa's advocacy for abstinence must be situated within a larger context in which scholars hotly debate the cause of Uganda's decline in HIV prevalence. Some studies report that a decrease in the average number of sexual partners, a later average age of sexual debut, and an increase in the number of youth reporting sexual abstinence have led to the decline in the HIV rate (Green 2003; Kiirya 1998; Green and Ruark 2008; Epstein 2007). Other studies have emphasized condom use and deaths from AIDS as factors contributing to the decrease (Gray et al. 2006; Wilson 2006). Comparing the studies' results, though, is problematic since they examine different time periods or regions of the country (Marshall 2008a). The complexity of the epidemic and the role of multiple factors in HIV rate decline provide opportunities for churches (and other AIDS organizations) to frame their AIDS efforts in numerous ways.

Churches with a Late, Broad Focus

Some churches in the final category began AIDS programs after the new millennium, while others had ad hoc AIDS efforts (such as pastoral counseling or congregational care committees) that they expanded after 2001. The Northmead Assembly of God Church in Lusaka, Zambia demonstrates this expansion into all six types of AIDS activities. Situated in a middle-class neighborhood, the congregation has over 2,000 members. It was started in 1971 by missionaries from the Pentecostal Assemblies of Canada Mission and until the late 1980s, it had only Western missionaries as pastors. Its pastor in 2010—Bishop Joshua Banda—came to the church in 1995. Increasingly approached by HIV-positive congregants for support and counseling during the late 1990s, Banda began to discuss AIDS indirectly, through a sermon series on death, dying, and grief. The church then began Bible study groups, during which nurses and doctors discussed the medical aspects of AIDS and other diseases. AIDS was not treated in isolation, partly to ease discussion of the topic and partly because HIV, TB, and malaria have high rates of co-infection. After several months of study, the congregation decided to provide HIV testing and counseling for its members. Its education efforts in the church and community have stressed sexual abstinence before marriage and marital fidelity. AIDS prevention activities also include HIV testing and counseling for singles, couples, and people who are going to get married (*Post*, June 5, 2005; FBO Roundtable 2009).

Support groups began when the pastor announced that anyone who was HIV-positive was invited to a meeting at his home. The "Circles of Hope" support organization formed in 2004 from the original seventeen congregants (sixteen women and one man) who attended the meeting. Groups of HIV-positive individuals began to meet regularly to share their struggles, concerns, and strategies for living well. Not only did the groups become a model for congregation-level spiritual outreach to HIV-positive Zambians (Ndhlovu 2007), but they also energized further AIDS program development in treatment and orphan care. As of 2007, the church provided ARVs to 1,800 people and care to roughly 3,800 individuals from the church and neighborhood. The church also has a care project for street children and children who were orphaned by AIDS (*Times of Zambia*, December 19, 2009). These efforts have helped to reduce stigma within the congregation and community. One church leader (Interview 7) explained that the church now talks openly about AIDS, because stigma and discrimination have been reduced. For example, there have been marriage ceremonies of HIV-positive church members in which the pastor openly refers to the couple's HIV status. These couples can be a model for living positively, demonstrating that "AIDS isn't the end of life."

Such discussions and activities created a foundation from which the church's pastor has gained an increasing role in national-level AIDS advocacy. Banda worked with other Zambian church leaders to form the Expanded Church Response to HIV/AIDS in 2000, a group with over two hundred church members. The organization works across denominations to initiate projects to build capacity for faith-based organizations and church-related health facilities, and to build the human capacity and social infrastructure of Zambia's Christian community (Expanded Church Response n.d.). The coalition has "given [churches] one thrust, and put them in a strategic place to do more than just building church capacity to respond. Instead we are in a place to do advocacy" (Interviews 7, 8; FBO Roundtable 2009). Political advocacy also is evident in Banda's participation in the National AIDS Council of Zambia since 2005. He has chaired several council committees and, during 2009, he served as the chairman of the entire council (FBO Roundtable 2009). In sum, the Northmead Assembly of God provides an example of a church involved in multiple AIDS activities, including political advocacy.

Making Sense of Church AIDS Activities

What factors influence the timing and scope of these church responses to AIDS? Using the explanatory variables of resources, state-church relations, and external factors, the next three chapters seek to answer that question. The chapters will utilize the abovementioned cases to illustrate larger themes, although at times, other church examples are included to provide a more complete analysis. Chapter 3 starts by questioning how resources shape church responses. I use three definitions of resources often touted by supporters of churches: biblical principles (or, a set of ideas that motivates action); organizational infrastructure; and pastoral leadership. I do not focus directly on financial resources, because interviewees did not stress this factor and because Chapter 5 analyzes finances from donors, who fund approximately 80 percent of Africa's AIDS programs. Chapter 3 asserts that the biblical themes (or frames) that churches emphasize shape the timing and scope of AIDS actions. The chapter argues that resources, particularly biblical interpretations and leadership, provide an important explanation for why some churches have done nothing on AIDS. I also assert that earlier responses capitalized on centralized church infrastructure, while later responses often relied on entrepreneurial pastors who designed new programs and built relationships with other churches, international faith-based organizations, and donors.

Chapter 4 investigates how state-church relations affect church AIDS actions. As discussed in Chapter 1, AIDS efforts are inherently political; they influence resource allocation and define social values. Additionally, many churches engage both directly and indirectly in the public realm. The chapter first examines how churches' past political involvement shapes AIDS efforts. Although it argues against path dependency, it finds that churches acting early on AIDS were those which had some previous political experiences and held a broad public theology that urged political involvement to foster justice.

I then look at how church participation in health care provision facilitated early and broad action on AIDS. As part of the church-state nexus, I examine opportunities for churches to participate in AIDS policy-making structures, particularly the Global Fund-required Country Coordinating Mechanisms. Because these entities were not established until 2003, their presence does not explain early actions on AIDS. However, I argue that representation on the Country Coordinating

Mechanisms can both reinforce (and bolster) early church efforts and urge later responses. Finally, the chapter situates church actions in a larger context of national political systems, religious competition, and state reactions to church AIDS activities. It asserts that context matters, but provides an incomplete explanation for why churches react as they do to AIDS.

Chapter 5 situates the timing and scope of African church AIDS actions in a global context. It investigates how external funding from USAID, the Global Fund, and PEPFAR affect church activities. Because the Global Fund and PEPFAR did not begin until after 2003, they could not have led some churches to initiate programs in the pre-2001 period, although USAID did provide support for some early church efforts. For many churches, AIDS action (or inaction) correlates with the availability of funding. However, the chapter argues that donor funding alone cannot explain church responses; global ecumenical bodies and networks influenced African church activities in both early and later periods.

The chapter also explores various levels of church agency in global collaboration. It finds that classifying churches as either impotent or independent is problematic. To demonstrate church agency, the chapter analyzes churches that challenge the international AIDS regime. Stephen Krasner (1982, 186) defines a regime as "implicit or explicit principles, norms, and decision-making procedures" that facilitate cooperation among actors. International organizations often play a role in facilitating the creation and maintenance of a regime's patterns of expectations and norms of behavior. Propagated by the World Health Organization, UNAIDS, public health experts, AIDS activists, and bilateral donors, the norms of the AIDS regime emphasize a biomedical approach based on known scientific facts. Notable among these facts are that the HIV virus causes AIDS; the virus can be transmitted from mother to child, through homosexual and heterosexual intercourse, and through tainted blood products and needles; AIDS has no known cure; and ARVs can decrease an infected person's viral load (Youde 2007; Iliffe 2006). This approach seeks technical means to decrease HIV transmission, such as comprehensive HIV education programs; education about and distribution of condoms; HIV prevention messages targeted to most-at-risk groups, such as men who have sex with men and commercial sex workers; HIV tests for pregnant women; a safe blood supply; provision of drugs to prevent mother-to-child transmission; and provision of clean needles for intravenous drug users (Iliffe 2006, 90). These policy prescriptions are also rooted in liberalism, or the belief that individuals should be free to make decisions about their sexual relations and that people can protect themselves from HIV if given adequate information, autonomy, and resources.

The final chapter asks what church involvement on AIDS will mean for African churches themselves and their long-term influence on Africa's other pressing health and development issues. It questions how the inactivity of some churches on AIDS shapes the ability of all churches to be legitimate actors on the issue. I situate these assessments in the context of a perceived decline in global concern about the pandemic in 2010. In doing so, I return to the book's introductory themes of the growth of African Christianity, churches as unique civil society actors, and donor attention to religion in international development.

---

[1] Conversation with author, Grand Rapids, Michigan, April 20, 2008.

[2] Recent research demonstrates the importance of church leaders in urging couples to participate in voluntary counseling and testing before marriage or pregnancy (Allen et al. 2007).

[3] AIDS experts debate whether formula or breastfeeding is better for babies of HIV-positive mothers. Since access to clean water and sterile bottles for formula feeding is difficult in much of Africa, formula feeding may prevent AIDS deaths but children may die of diarrhea. While initially the World Health Organization and UNICEF advised against breastfeeding for HIV-positive mothers, recent studies have shown that the risk of HIV transmission comes mainly from the combination of breast milk and other foods, such as formula and solids. The combination can damage the baby's intestines, inviting infection. In a study in Botswana, breast-fed babies contracted HIV at a higher rate, but formula-fed babies were more likely to die. If the mother is on ARV treatment, the risk of mother-to-child transmission through breastfeeding declines to 2 percent (*Washington Post*, July 23, 2007, A1).

[4] Author observations at meeting with home-based care church group, Lusaka, Zambia, August 11, 2007.

[5] Notable exceptions were Presidents Yoweri Museveni of Uganda and Abdou Diouf of Senegal. Similarly, several high-level religious leaders in those two countries spoke about the disease.

[6] In a cursory examination of the websites for ten American-based, Christian development organizations, nine of the ten concentrated their efforts in Anglophone countries. The one exception was Catholic Relief Services, which has stronger links to Francophone countries because the Catholic Church is more active than Protestant churches in those countries. The ten organizations include World Vision International (http://www.wvi.org), Compassion International (http://www.compassion.com), Feed the Hungry (http://www.feedthehungry.org), Samaritan's Purse (http://www.samaritanspurse.org), Partners Worldwide (http://www.partnersworldwide.org), Mennonite Central Committee (http://mcc.org), World Concern (http://www.worldconcern.org), MAP International (http://www.map.org), Food for the Hungry (http://www.fh.org), and Catholic Relief Services (http://crs.org). While I also investigated Christian

Children's Fund, now called ChildFund International (http://www.ChildFund.org), the absence of any mention of Christianity led me to exclude the organization from this analysis. I do not claim this list is inclusive of all Christian development organizations in the United States.

[7] Author conversation at the Network of African Congregational Theology Conference on AIDS, Poverty, and the Church in Africa, Lusaka, Zambia, August 7, 2007 (see also Botha 2007; Mhungu 2007).

[8] As of 2009, the fifteen denominations included the African Methodist Episcopal Church, the African Methodist Episcopal Zion Church, Christ Evangelical Mission, Christian Methodist Episcopal Church, Eden Revival Church, International Evangelical Church of Ghana, Evangelical Lutheran Church of Ghana, Ghana Baptist Convention, Ghana Mennonite Church, Greek Orthodox Church, Methodist Church Ghana, Presbyterian Church of Ghana, Religious Society of Friends, the Salvation Army, and Evangelical Presbyterian Church, Ghana. The two organizational members were the Young Men's Christian Association (YMCA) and the Young Women's Christian Association (YWCA).

[9] The US Congress first approved money for prevention of mother-to-child transmission in select African countries in 2002, although these programs did not fully scale up until PEPFAR's passage in 2003 (*New York Times*, June 20, 2002).

[10] Information on the African Jesuits AIDS Network is available at http://www.jesuitsaids.net.

[11] Information about Ssempa's speaking schedule can be found on his personal website. See http://www.martinssempa.com.

[12] Uganda's HIV rate increased slightly to 5.4 percent in 2007 (UNAIDS 2009e).

3
Resources and Choices

Both the civil society and social movement literatures assert that resources are crucial for effective and legitimate mobilization to address social and political issues (van Stekelenburg and Klandermans 2009; Patterson 2006; McCarthy and Zald 1977; Gyimah-Boadi 2004). While the civil society literature tends to focus on tangible resources such as funding and human capacity, these are not the only assets churches have (Marshall 2008a). Many church interviewees recognized their organizations lacked financial resources; for them, Africa's poor economic development meant other resources were crucial determinants of the timing and scope of church AIDS actions (Interviews 1, 2, 9, 10, 23, 29, 47, 49, 51). Biblical principles that helped to frame the disease, church organizational structures, and pastoral leadership emerged as drivers of AIDS mobilization.[1] This chapter explicates the role of these three. It acknowledges that although churches may resemble civil society groups in many ways, their focus on biblical frameworks sets them apart from secular associations.

I begin with an examination of biblical themes as a resource for framing activities. Because individuals vary greatly in the ways they perceive problems, frame alignment is a necessary process for any type of social mobilization. As schemata for interpreting situations and mobilizing action, frames develop through dynamic and interactional processes. Frames may compete and change over time. Frame alignment includes what Snow et al. (1986) term frame amplification (i.e., clarifying and interpreting a frame) and frame transformation (i.e., expanding a frame to encompass broader issues). While I use the social movement concept of frame and the term biblical concept to delineate ideas that motivate church actions, I hesitate to use the term theology in reference to church understandings of AIDS. A theology is a comprehensive, biblically-derived worldview that provides a larger template for understanding the nature of God, religious experiences, and the physical and spiritual realms. In many cases, churches adopt seemingly contradictory stances on HIV and AIDS, making it difficult to argue that they have a coherent theology about the disease. For example, a church may proclaim that God made human beings to be a part of a religious community, but then refuse to baptize or marry parishioners living with HIV.

To explain the various stances adopted by churches, I focus on four Christian concepts that frame church mobilization: (1) AIDS as God's punishment for sin; (2) biblical rules for living a moral life; (3) God's power to heal disease as demonstrated directly and indirectly through the life of God's son Jesus Christ; and (4) Jesus Christ's love and compassion for all people, because they are made in God's image.[2] While these messages can be derived from biblical principles the first two are more prevalent in the Hebrew Bible and the latter two in the New Testament.[3] Churches that have either not acted to fight AIDS or have acted narrowly tend to focus more on the themes of God's punishment for sin and his rules for so-called moral living (Interviews 33, 49).[4] The belief in God's power to heal also motivates the narrowly focused spiritual healing efforts. In contrast, the themes of Jesus Christ's acceptance and care for marginalized people and the belief that God created humans in his image have tended to influence churches with early and more comprehensive efforts.

The chapter then examines organizational resources as a determinant of the timing and scope of church actions. Civil society scholars have paid only limited attention to organizational structures and internal decision making processes for both religious and secular organizations. Yet, the structure of an organization can positively or negatively influence internal communication, decision making, and accountability (Patterson 1998; Fatton 1995). These issues are no less apparent in churches, where divisions between leaders and rank-and-file members may negatively affect church legitimacy and effectiveness (Chitando 2007; Englund 2000). I define organizational resources in two ways: church hierarchy and participation in coalitions. I argue that hierarchical churches were able to act more quickly and comprehensively to address AIDS since this structure facilitated exchange of information and rapid implementation of decisions. In contrast, more decentralized churches acted more recently, if at all, to combat the disease. I also assert that coalitions were not an impetus for early actions on AIDS, but may help sustain later activities.

The third section maintains that in addition to being crucial social and spiritual leaders throughout Africa, pastors have played a particularly central role in urging church efforts on AIDS after 2001. While pastors have always been well respected, I focus here on their increased managerial and entrepreneurial skills, particularly among African Pentecostal churches. (These include the more established and the newer Pentecostal churches.) As Pentecostalism has grown, some churches have become less egalitarian and decentralized in their structures and more hierarchical and pastor-centered (Kalu 2008). I maintain that some of these churches were uniquely situated to capitalize on recent global interest in the disease, because their pastors have media ministries, large followings, more educational training than in past generations, and often, relations with American evangelical churches. These pastors have used both public events and private networking through small church groups to urge both narrow and broad AIDS mobilization.

Biblical Principles that Motivate Actions on AIDS

As several interviewees explained, most African churches lack a comprehensive theology with which to understand AIDS. Moreover, there is not even agreement among churches about the need for such a doctrine (Interviews 2, 25, 47, 53, 55). At the ecumenical level, there have been some attempts to develop such a theology, such as the Ecumenical Advocacy Alliance's 2005-2008 Framework for Action and its 2009 book on biblical principles and HIV prevention (Paterson 2009; Ecumenical Advocacy Alliance 2005). Some African theologians have written extensively on the pandemic (Dube 2002; Haddad 2002; West 2003; Chitando 2007; Schmid 2006; Bongmba 2007; Katongole 2005). Many of their ideas have been disseminated through the World Council of Churches and through Catholic bishops, and many are available online. Yet, given the general lack of resources for African churches and seminaries, and many pastors' isolation from internet access and continued pastoral education, these resources often do not reach those who need them.[5]

The lack of an overarching framework on AIDS has prevented some churches from designing long-term, comprehensive AIDS programs, sustaining initial efforts, and fostering a public voice on the disease (Interview 2; Bongmba 2007; Chitando 2007). As with social movement actors who may have different or competing frames for mobilization, the lack of coherence among churches on AIDS leads to various church AIDS responses. Individual churches have tended to stress particular biblical themes to frame their own approaches to the disease. While most churches and Christians understand the world's issues in terms of multiple biblical principles, churches may emphasize specific scriptural themes to situate their specific approaches to the disease. To simplify this analysis, I treat the following biblical themes independently, although they may inform one another.

God's Punishment for Sin and His Rules for Holy Living

Framing AIDS mobilization in punitive language, some churches rely on a literal reading of biblical texts against promiscuity, prostitution, and homosexuality, particularly the story of God's destruction of Sodom and Gomorrah (Haddad 2005).[6] These texts not only set rules for moral living, but they also demonstrate that an omnipotent God punishes those who sin against him with death. Because HIV infection and AIDS lead to death, particularly among young people who should otherwise be healthy, these churches view the disease to be the result of sin (Mukuka and Slonim-Nevo 2006; Garner 2000b; Paterson 2001, 2). This perspective asserts that God is a deity who demands justice, or some type of retribution for transgressions; God wills the punishments of death, eternal condemnation, and/or isolation from the religious community for people who are infected with HIV (Czerny and Vitillo 2005-2006, 277).

The "God-as-punisher" viewpoint has caused some churches to ignore the disease in their congregations because they do not want to interfere with God's plan for "sinners" (Interviews 30, 35, 36, 49). Some churches may argue that ignoring, stigmatizing, and ostracizing HIV-positive Christians is a part of God's plan, because when God punished sinners in the Hebrew Bible, he often drove them from the community (Garner 2000b).[7] Fear of this church reaction leads individuals to hide their HIV-positive status. One Ghanaian AIDS educator explained about a prominent church leader, "He says he would never disclose his status to his church, because he has seen how people in the community react to those with the disease and the ways their children are treated" (Interview 29). Similar stories are common in other countries (Parry 2003; WCC 2001; Interviews 1, 2, 9, 14, 16).

However, not all churches that emphasize that AIDS results from sinful actions shun, ostracize, or ignore HIV-positive people. Some focus on educating people to follow God's commands because "AIDS results from not living a moral life" (Interview 33). One pastor in Ghana explained, "Even if we do not see AIDS as punishment for sin or AIDS as sin, we can still see that it is sinful to abuse our bodies. And we can see that sexual immorality is against God" (Interview 37).

These churches condemn sex before marriage, multiple sexual partners, sexual relations outside of marriage, homosexuality, and prostitution. They point to the explicit rules for "holy living" outlined in

Leviticus 18 and commands about marital commitment found throughout the Bible.[8] Many, but not all, of these churches are Pentecostal, and they stress the need for a holiness ethic for all believers (Kalu 2008, 19). For these churches, there is "no compromise on immorality" (Interview 37), and they believe that progress on AIDS can only occur when society reforms its behavior. One pastor explained: "The AIDS cure isn't in sight now because God detests immorality. Until behavior changes, HIV/AIDS won't change" (Interview 31). Catholics and mainline Protestants also incorporate morality messages, as southern African Catholic bishops did in 2006 when they stressed that morality is the only "true, sustainable solution" to the disease (*Catholic Information Service for Africa*, November 21, 2006). Yet, these two types of churches are more likely to situate these commands in a framework of comprehensive AIDS efforts. In contrast, churches with the narrow morality focus tend to concentrate their programs on HIV prevention.

Since youth are often the target audience for these prevention messages, these churches have paid less attention to prevention through marital fidelity, although this is changing in some countries. Given the fact that sex with multiple concurrent partners is an avenue for HIV transmission, and that marital faithfulness is a biblical theme, one might assume churches would place greater emphasis on this prevention message (Epstein 2007).[9] However, as several African theologians have pointed out (Haddad 2002; Chitando 2007), some church leaders may lack credibility on this issue because of their own involvement in extra-marital relations. One interviewee explained,

> Pastors may preach the be-faithful message, but they are sometimes the problem. You go to church and the pastor preaches abstinence or faithfulness, but you know about their relationships. And I think, 'Who are you deceiving?' We are really lacking in role models. (Interview 35)[10]

While moral messages have always been part of the churches' approach to AIDS, this theme has gotten more media attention and response from donors in recent years (Iliffe 2006). The large amount of global coverage that Ssempa's abstinence messages have gained illustrates this point (Epstein 2007; Blumenthal 2009; Ssempa 2005; Ssempa 2009). This attention to morality should be placed in a context in which church leaders perceive that a liberal, biomedical approach to AIDS dominates, particularly with its focus on condom distribution. One church official explained:

> Christians do not accept a defeatist [liberal] message that people cannot abstain [from sex] and thus, we should just give the youth condoms. Some AIDS groups say Christians are just hypocrites for acting like they can abstain. But acceptance of condoms defeats the Gospel of Christ [or the belief that with God's help, believers can repent of sinful behavior]. (Interview 30)

From the perspective of the pastor (and others who share his views), the fight against AIDS is not about condom distribution or ARV treatment, but rather it is about "doing the right thing," or abstaining from sex before marriage or outside of committed monogamous heterosexual relationships (Ssempa 2009).

Some church leaders and members have linked the emphasis on sexual morality to ARV treatment programs. They assert that because ARVs make HIV-positive people look and feel healthy, these HIV-positive people may not act responsibly in their sexual relationships. Instead, these individuals will engage in pre-marital sex, sex with multiple partners, or sex outside of marriage. This fear has caused a minority of church leaders and members (from all types of churches) to be wary of ARVs (Msoka 2009; Kalipeni, Muula, and Liwewe 2009).

In contrast, a few churches have sought to situate support for condoms in the morality framework. One church AIDS coordinator explained:

> Pastors say that condoms are only 85 percent effective, [but this is] an excuse to not discuss them. And we'd say, yes, but 85 percent is better than nothing. And wouldn't you rather keep [your parishioners] alive with the 85 percent so that they can sit in church and listen to your sermons where you talk about morality and behavior change? Wouldn't you like to keep them alive, so that they have the opportunity to change their behavior? (Interview 35)

Other religious and secular AIDS educators explained that it was moral to help people live and thus, condoms play a role in fighting AIDS (Interviews 2, 38, 43). Despite such attempts, churches opposed to condoms have usually been unwilling to re-evaluate their views in light of such moral claims.

There is considerable debate among activists, public health workers, and churches about how the focus on moral living (defined as abstinence and marital fidelity) shapes the fight against AIDS. While abstinence and fidelity within relationships where each partner has the same sero-status prevent new HIV infections, some activists, public health experts, and church officials fear that the emphasis on morality increases the disease's stigma (Krakauer and Newbery 2007; Epstein 2007).[11] For this reason, some church efforts (such as Ghana's Compassion Campaign) have sought to de-emphasize morality: "[We wanted people to know] AIDS had nothing to do with morality and everything to do with a mistake, just one mistake" (Interview 35). The morality framework also downplays the economic, social, cultural, and psychological reasons why people (particularly women, migrants, and the poor) may engage in sex before marriage or with multiple partners. Some argue that the sexual morality perspective has the danger of emphasizing individual agency while forgetting cultural and structural challenges, as when a Ugandan bishop blamed the country's epidemic on the generosity of female Christians: "They give in to useless men, allowing them to play with their bodies" (*New Vision*, February 2, 2006). Such statements, it is feared, further drive HIV-positive people from the church, and more broadly, prevent them from accessing services for people living with HIV/AIDS (Interviews 29, 36, 60).

God's Power to Heal

According to the Bible, the God who punishes sinners can also heal physical and mental ailments. Stories of medical miracles are dispersed throughout the Bible: God reportedly made the elderly Sarai pregnant and cured Naaman's leprosy, while Jesus Christ healed people with severe pains, seizures, and paralysis.[12] One Pentecostal pastor explained, "God has a cure for AIDS, otherwise he would not have said he was the healer of every disease." For this pastor, however, the cure would come when God was ready to reveal it (Interview 31). Churches apply belief in God's healing power to their AIDS efforts in different ways. For many churches, this power is evident in the development of ARVs which, while they do not kill HIV, have made the infection manageable (Interview 60; FBO Roundtable 2009).

A smaller number of churches believe that God cures HIV and AIDS through a spiritual battle with the evil forces that have brought HIV infection. (Some of these churches acknowledge the scientific evidence for the virus; others do not.) This spiritual healing is situated in an African cosmology that stresses the belief that for every disease or misfortune, there is a larger spiritual cause. This framework divides illness into either physical or spiritual sicknesses. The former have physical causes and biomedical cures, while the latter result from supernatural causes, such as personal or communal sins, the breach of religious taboos, or the activities of evil powers such as witches.[13] Some individuals with this perspective assert that powerful, wealthy individuals who contract HIV have been punished for their sins of corruption; others believe that all of African society is paying through the AIDS pandemic for the evil actions of a corrupt few (Iliffe 2006; Ellis and ter Haar 2004). Supernatural causes often are used to explain traumatic, mysterious, and abnormal situations, such as accidents or deaths of the very young. Because AIDS deaths fall into this category, churches that view AIDS through a "healing" framework try to invoke spiritual power to cure the disease (Asamoah-Gyadu 2005b). Healers communicate with the spiritual realm through prayer and then use their spiritual power to exorcise HIV from the infected person through strategies such as hard labor, fasting, carrying heavy loads, beating, or even forced sexual relations (Kwansa 2009; *Daily Graphic*, September 25, 2008).

As Ellis and ter Haar (2004) point out, since governments were relatively silent about their country's AIDS epidemics until after 2001, the vacuum in public discussion was filled with common understandings of illness and death. In societies where poor people lack access to biomedical health care, spiritual healing is an attractive alternative. Birgit Meyer (1998) finds that most members of one Ghanaian Pentecostal church joined the congregation precisely for the possible healing it might provide. Spiritual healing also may provide hope in a context where the disease has no cure and ARV access remains limited: "If man has failed, then you can come to God and have something from him, what man cannot provide" (Tanzanian pastor, quoted in Dilger 2007, 69). Healing pastors and their congregations are accessible, particularly with the rise of Pentecostalism across Africa. Spiritual healing also may help the person with HIV come to terms with the larger emotional questions that ARV treatment cannot address, such as "Why me?"

On the other hand, spiritual healing can complicate ARV treatment programs, hasten the death of those with AIDS, foster false hope, destroy the religious faith of HIV-positive people, and contribute to society's denial of the disease. Those who undergo exorcism through hard labor, chaining, flogging, or fasting may become quite ill. In Ghana, a country with over five hundred prayer camps in which journalists report that "flagrant human rights abuses… are a daily phenomena," there are many stories of HIV-positive individuals dying in camp healing efforts (*Daily Graphic*, September 25, 2008).[14] A Zambian AIDS activist further explained the difficulty of merging spiritual healing with ARV treatment:

> Some [charismatic] churches are telling people they are healed; they don't need to take their drugs. But if people go off treatment, it is hard to bring them back into the treatment regimen. They think, 'I've been healed.' So even if they get sick, they won't go back on treatment, because the prominent authority figure—the pastor—has told them they were healed and they believed in this healing. Our AIDS group has lost several members [to death] because of this. (Banda 2009)

Spiritual healing has given rise to a contingent of charlatan healers who create false hope for HIV-positive people who are emotionally and physically vulnerable. One Kampala pastor blackmailed and bribed worshippers to fake health problems such as AIDS so that she could claim to cure them (*Monitor*, October 9, 2007). When pastors cannot cure AIDS, the person with the disease is often blamed for a lack of faith or devotion or for not giving adequate financial resources to the church. Such accusations can destroy the religious faith of the person, often at the stage in the illness when the person most needs support, love, and care from a faith community. One leader of an ecumenical organization explained, "There are lots of people in these churches bearing a lot of pain [when they are not cured and told that they do not have enough faith to be cured]. Often this pain means leaving. But, they aren't just leaving these individual churches; they are leaving the church altogether and that is a tragedy" (Interview 53). Some critics also assert that by denying the scientific fact that AIDS cannot be cured, these churches are complicit in denial of the disease (Banda 2009).

The line between biomedical treatment and spiritual healing is blurry, and for many individuals living with HIV/AIDS, there is a dynamic process by which they come to terms with the spiritual-biomedical tension. One Zambian physician explained that many people come to the doctor's AIDS clinic after seeking healing with traditional medicines or from Pentecostal healing ceremonies. When the people arrive, they still believe that God will cure them. The doctor described the clinic's response, and the patients' changed perspective:

> We tell them that the Lord gives us [ARV] treatment to treat the disease. He gives us medicine. We tell them that we believe in miracles too. But for us scientific laws lead to the benefits of healing and medicine. And we see that over time, they believe in the medicine too. The medicine is their miracle, because they come to us, get the treatment, and they get better. (Interview 60)

In summary, the sole focus on spiritual healing has led to a narrow approach to AIDS. Pastors and Christian AIDS workers such as the

Zambian physician have sought to put healing into a broader context of biomedical explanations for the disease and they have tended to address AIDS more comprehensively. As the next section illustrates, they have also relied on other biblical principles to frame their actions.

Christ's Care, Acceptance, and Love for All of God's Image Bearers

In the New Testament, Jesus Christ directs his followers to care for the homeless, hungry, sick, and lonely people in society. He explains that believers who have not cared for "the least of these" will receive "eternal punishment."[15] Jesus emphasizes that every human being is entitled to care when he tells the story of the Good Samaritan. The Samaritan, a member of a group despised and distrusted in Hebrew society, provides shelter, food, and care for the beaten and robbed stranger the Samaritan encounters on the road, while the Hebrew priests and teachers ignore the person in need.[16] Christ's emphasis on compassion serves as the foundation for churches that have a comprehensive approach to AIDS. Part of this comprehensive approach may include urging abstinence and faithfulness, although this message is often conveyed through a paradigm of Christian love, rather than a rubric of "dos and don'ts." A Lutheran missionary in Uganda explains, "The secret of teaching is that you can't scream at people… you have to use a special approach. I call it love. If people really feel you care for them, you can be quite open" (quoted in Epstein 2007, 200).

Christian compassion can lead to a more holistic approach to health and development, one which is also rooted in the belief that God created people in his image and desires for them to live in community. If one individual is hurting, the entire community suffers (Bongmba 2007, 46). The bonds between God and his creation (human beings) can never be broken, even though humans may turn from God. Because they are created in God's image, people are complex creatures who are not defined solely by their physical bodies, emotions, or social positions. This theological concept, summed up in the Latin phrase *imago dei*, particularly informed the early and comprehensive work of the Catholic Church. More recently, though, this emphasis on holistic development is evident in some Pentecostal churches with broader efforts on AIDS (Miller and Yamamori 2007).

The emphasis on Christian compassion and the *imago dei* provides a transformative frame for church mobilization. Frame transformation moves the AIDS issue beyond a narrow discussion of sexual morality or spiritual healing to encompass themes such as poverty or Christian community. Frame transformation has caused some churches to argue that Christians who stigmatize or shun people living with HIV/AIDS are demonizing God, since all people bear some resemblance to him (Bongmba 2007). Instead of emphasizing the view that God punishes people living with HIV/AIDS, these churches often compare individuals with the disease to stigmatized groups in the New Testament with whom Jesus interacted, such as lepers, the disabled, adulterers, sex workers, and tax collectors.[17] Jesus challenges a crowd that is about to stone a woman caught in adultery: "If anyone of you is without sin, let him be the first to throw a stone at her."[18] This command to withhold judgment informed the Compassion Campaign in Ghana with its slogan: "Who are you to judge?" It also led some churches, such as the Anglican Church in Kenya, to apologize for their early attitudes toward people living with HIV/AIDS: "As a Church, our earlier approach in fighting AIDS was misplaced, since we likened it to a disease for sinners and a curse from God. We apologise [*sic*] for earlier abandoning our flock" (*Daily Telegraph*, March 18, 2006).

An acknowledgement of the complexity of the human condition pushes churches with the comprehensive approach to address the disease holistically with programs to meet the physical, emotional, community, mental, and spiritual needs of people living with HIV/AIDS (Parry 2003; Bongmba 2007). While this is most evident in the Catholic programs that combine treatment access, nutritional support for those on ARVs, care for those who are sick, and employment, education, and housing support for people infected with or affected by HIV/AIDS, in recent years some Protestant organizations have taken up this holistic approach.[19] One Catholic AIDS worker explained about why treatment and food distribution must go together: "The Bible tells us to pray for our daily bread" (Fikansa 2009). Another church AIDS coordinator commented that spiritual support is not sufficient for those living with the disease:

> Of course, we do spiritual counseling, but people cannot live by the spirit alone. The church is not just about spiritual issues; it also about the material conditions of life. If we cannot help people to live better lives, then spiritual salvation doesn't matter. (Interview 41)

This holistic understanding of AIDS is sometimes framed in the language of morality. That is, some churches assert that as moral agents, they should provide food, shelter, care, support, medicines, and prayer, not only commands to live a "sexually disciplined life." This type of moral frame transformation has been most explicitly used to argue for provision of ARV treatment to Africans (Friedman and Mottiar 2004;

Newsweek, February 18, 2002). Despite such efforts, either because of media coverage or conventional wisdom, the "morality message" has tended to be defined more narrowly in terms of sexual morality, not the larger provision of services and support, a point which frustrates some churches with a more holistic approach to AIDS and which limits broader mobilization efforts (FBO Roundtable 2009).

In reality, even churches that emphasize the *imago dei* have difficulty fully applying the concept's implications to the disease. As one HIV-positive person said, when a church member looks at people with HIV or AIDS they have a hard time "seeing God in our image" (Banda 2009). Since Africans stress a powerful God, or a God who created the world and fights demons, and they do not emphasize the suffering of God through the crucifixion of Jesus Christ, the idea that a weak and disfigured person is God-like is difficult to comprehend (Omenyo 2008; Banda 2009).

An additional challenge of the holistic approach is that many churches are uncomfortable viewing sexuality as part of the complex human identity. Despite the fact that several Catholic and Protestant documents on AIDS make this point,[20] few churches want to talk about "sex as a gift from God" (FBO Roundtable 2009). One Reformed Church pastor in Zambia described how he almost lost his job when he preached on sexuality (Ndhlovu 2007, 164-165). Another Ghanaian church leader explained that pastors did not think it was appropriate to discuss sex in public, particularly with youth (Interview 30). It was the rare pastor who discussed sex openly and framed sex as something God created (FBO Roundtable 2009). Another extension of the *imago dei* theme would be for churches to situate AIDS in the context of the structural variables of poverty, patriarchy, and domestic violence that make people vulnerable to HIV infection (Kelly 2007; Interviews 2, 23; Chitando 2007). Few churches, regardless of the scope or timing of their AIDS activities, have extended their efforts to this level.

To be clear, all churches still struggle with the idea that it is not just people "outside the body of Christ" who live with HIV and AIDS (Interview 1), a fact which continues to limit the development of a common framework for mobilization. Nevertheless, biblical principles, although not always coherent, have helped to shape the breadth and timing of church actions. Church inaction is rooted in the view that the disease is a punishment for sin. While influential for all churches, biblical rules about holy living shape more recent, narrow approaches to AIDS. The belief that AIDS results from evil spirits and can only be cured through exorcism, prayers, traditional herbs, and/or cleansing may lead some churches to narrowly focus on spiritual healing. In contrast, the *imago dei* concept and the model of Christ's compassion foster a more comprehensive approach to the disease that takes into account the holistic nature of the human condition. The idea that only God (not other sinful believers) can judge urged some churches to act early and broadly to fight AIDS.

Even though church leaders may frame AIDS in light of particular biblical themes, church members may view the epidemic very differently. This tension can negatively influence programs to combat HIV and AIDS. For example, pastors may urge compassion, while members continue to stigmatize people living with HIV/AIDS (Kwansa 2009). This disconnect seems less apparent in high prevalence countries. Zambian Christian leaders and congregants talked about Jesus Christ's compassion for the sick. One official with a faith-based organization that works with 11,000 Zambian home-based care volunteers reported: "If you ask the volunteers why they do the home-based care, 90 percent of the time, they say, 'It's my Christian calling to love my neighbor'" (Interview 12). On the other hand, the leader-follower disconnect may have partly prevented long-run, high-level action on the disease by Ghanaian churches after the Compassion Campaign ended. While church leaders advocated frames of Christian compassion and the *imago dei*, rank-and-file members were more likely to approach the disease from the "spiritual curse" and the narrow "moral behavior" perspectives (Interviews 35, 36, 46, 47, 51). For many Ghanaian church members, AIDS remained a disease that only infected non-Christians. If leaders wanted to discuss the epidemic, church members had little interest. One Christian AIDS worker explained about his efforts to educate youth: "It can get to the point where the issue is 'repulsive' to them. . . . We were going to do a program on AIDS and show a film, and one person said, 'This is too much. We are always talking about AIDS'" (Interview 36). In such a situation, the leader-member divide and the lack of a common identity rooted in a shared frame for understanding AIDS may prevent the church from effectively addressing the disease.

Organizational Resources

Social scientists within the new institutionalist paradigm point to the ways rules and structures affect political and social outcomes (March and Olsen 1989; Firmin-Sellers 1995; Moe 1990). While they often focus on formal structures, their insights help explain how (or if) civil society organizations can effectively meet their goals or make decisions that are viewed to be legitimate among their members (Patterson 2003; Putnam 1994). In the case of religious associations, Carolyn Warner and

Manfred Wenner (2006) find that the organizational structures of Islam partially explain why Muslim believers in Western Europe have had limited involvement in politics. Here I am concerned with how two elements of church organization—hierarchy and participation in various types of coalitions—influence the timing and breadth of church AIDS responses. As I examine coalitions, I will pay particular attention to the ways that Christian involvement in these coalitions may affect other religious groups such as Muslims and adherents of African traditional religions. I also will examine the ways that people living with HIV/AIDS are encouraged to collaborate with churches.

My definition of organizational resources puts aside questions about church members' religious devotion or socioeconomic backgrounds, or the church's location. Because congregants' assumed spiritual commitment and loyalty to the church exist to a certain extent in all churches, these qualities cannot explain *variation* in church AIDS efforts. Similarly, even though churches with more activities tend to be located in urban areas and to have middle class congregations, these membership characteristics do not explicate the timing and scope of those churches' actions.

I also do not define organizational resources as capacity, or the ability of an organization (or the state) to meet its objectives (Englebert 2000). Because monetary resources, leadership, and membership size affect capacity, it is difficult to examine capacity in isolation. The interviews revealed that almost all churches claim to "lack capacity," a fact which decreased the power of this explanation for why churches differ in the timing and scope of their AIDS activities. Leaders of comprehensive, lengthy AIDS programs cited a lack of capacity, as did pastors of churches without any AIDS efforts (Interviews 1, 9, 10, 14, 16, 17, 27, 45, 50, 53).[21] Additionally, leaders of religious organizations defined low capacity in various ways. Some said low capacity means the organization lacks staff members to collect scientific, empirical evidence to support their advocacy or to monitor and evaluate AIDS programs (Interviews 9, 10, 14, 16, 17). Others reported that churches may have personnel, but these staff members are inadequately educated about AIDS or the scientific changes in ARV treatment (Interviews 36, 46). Personnel get tired ("burned out") with the issue (Interviews 26, 43), and because of morbidity and mortality, the disease itself limits the institutional memory of churches. AIDS kills pastors, church leaders, and seminary students (Banda 2007; Interviews 9, 10). While these effects should not be discounted, they influence all churches. Thus, the organizational approach used here concentrates on how church hierarchy and church involvement in coalitions shapes the timing and scope of AIDS efforts.

Hierarchy and Church Structures

Churches can be placed on a continuum of most-to-least hierarchical, with the Catholic Church being the most and some Old Independents and smaller New Independents, the least. The doctrine of papal infallibility places the Pope at the top of Catholic decision making, and the Vatican's overall policies (such as on human rights, the death penalty, or contraception) inform the actions of all Catholic institutions. Vatican priorities shape the policy directives that national and regional ecclesiastical conferences of bishops make. These directives then are passed down from the dioceses to individual parishes. As in any hierarchical organization, the local implementation of these directives can vary widely. Bishops at the diocesan level make many day-to-day administrative decisions about personnel and budgets. This hierarchical organization makes it easier for the church to act as a unified actor. In the political realm, unity makes it more likely the church will achieve its goals in its interactions with the state (Manuel, Reardon, and Wilcox 2007, 3).

Despite this hierarchy, there is country and historical variation in the involvement of the Catholic Church on socioeconomic and political issues. For example, Malawi's bishops challenged the authoritarian ruler Hastings Banda in a pastoral letter in March 1992 (Newell 1995). In contrast, the bishops of Rwanda ignored the genocide, and some priests actively participated in killings (Rutagambwa 2007, 178-180; Longman 2010). In Angola, the Catholic Church changed its position on injustice over time, from defense of Portuguese colonialism to post-independence demands for peace negotiations in the country's long war (Heywood 2007). Thus, while hierarchical, the Catholic Church is not homogeneous or static.

On the other end of the hierarchical spectrum are many of the Old Independent churches, particularly the smaller ones in rural areas, and some of the Pentecostal churches. Yet, it is important to recognize that Pentecostals vary greatly, and while many congregations may have local autonomy from other churches, there can be considerable hierarchy within individual congregations. For the New Independent churches, a dynamic pastor, who is "eloquent and persuasive in speech," often is the founder of the church, and power and decision making revolve around that person (Sackey 2006, 34). Established Pentecostal churches, such as the Assemblies of God or Apostolic Faith Church which are part of larger denominations introduced by Western missionaries, have more ties to those denominations but still allow a high level of autonomy in congregational decision making (US Assemblies of God 2009; Apostolic Faith Church 2009).[22] For most Pentecostal churches, individual congregations make decisions about programs and personnel, and they often are self-sufficient in financing.

In recent years, some Pentecostal churches have experienced tensions in their internal structures. In one sense, Pentecostalism emphasizes the idea of a "priesthood of all believers" which stresses that church members can participate in decision making and asserts that anyone (including women) who is "called by the Spirit" can become a pastor or church leader (Sackey 2006; Kalu 2008, 137). These beliefs may foster equality and democratic participation within autonomous church organizations (Patterson 2005; Miller and Yamamori 2007). On the other hand, the growth in Pentecostalism and the rise of urban mega-churches in the last generation have necessitated that churches become more internally hierarchical to facilitate efficiency, uniformity, and communication. While congregations may remain somewhat autonomous from other churches in a denomination, they are increasingly hierarchical in their own decision-making processes. Central to these new structures is the congregation's pastor, who may reinforce his (or sometimes, her) status with a university degree or advanced theological training, facilitated by the growth of Pentecostal universities and seminaries such as the Church of God Redeemer University in Nigeria (Akanji 2009; Omenyo 2008; Kalu 2008, 138).

Some Pentecostal pastors run large organizations; the church may own media outlets to televise its worship services; it may hire many staff members; it may own property such as auditoriums, offices, and primary schools. Some pastors resemble the "heads of giant institutions that employ staff that are comparable, if not bigger, to some … companies" (*Daily Graphic*, November 20, 2008). This hierarchy became apparent when a student researcher and I attempted to interview someone about AIDS programs at International Central Gospel Church, a neo-Pentecostal church in central Accra with over 7,000 attendees on a typical Sunday (Gifford 2004, 24). The behemoth organization, with its huge staff, maze-like building, "minders" to guide us, and multiple and confusing lines of communication, made arranging a conversation difficult. As I argue below, these relatively recent changes in Pentecostal structures, as well as the rise of more educated and cosmopolitan Pentecostal pastors, have implications for church AIDS actions.

The Old Mission Protestant Churches (that is, the mainline Protestants) tend to fall in the middle of the hierarchy continuum, with some such as the Anglicans exhibiting more hierarchy and ties to the larger global Anglican community, and some, like the Baptists, being more congregational. For example, the Presbyterian Church, a denomination prevalent in Anglophone countries, allows congregations to make decisions about budgetary priorities, personnel, and local programs (South African Presbyterian Church 2009). At the same time, representatives who are pastors and lay leaders chosen from local congregations make broad policies (such as rules for ordination of pastors or acceptance of creedal statements that outline theological beliefs) for the entire denomination. Pastors in the mainline Protestant denominations tend to be relatively well educated, often in the schools established by colonial missionaries (Gifford 1998).

Another aspect of the Old and New Mission Protestant Churches is that they tend to be linked together in ecumenical bodies, such as the Christian Council of Ghana (Old Mission Protestants) or the Evangelical Fellowship of Zambia (New Mission Protestants). Some of the Old Independent Churches such as the African Methodist Episcopal Zionists have joined national ecumenical councils, but many have not. More recently, some of the New Independent churches have formed such associations (Barrett and Johnson 2004).While these ecumenical bodies do not make decisions for their various denominational members, they do coordinate action and represent their members' interests in the political realm. The national-level ecumenical bodies for the mainline churches have long histories (most were started before independence), and thus, considerable experience in advocacy, policy negotiations, and program development (Gifford 1998).

Given the great variation in church structures, how has hierarchy affected the timing and scope of church efforts to fight AIDS? In general, hierarchy facilitated and helped to sustain the Catholic Church's early actions on AIDS. More broadly, the Catholic hierarchy, resources, and organization made it possible for the Catholic Church to be one of the most powerful (if not the most powerful) social institutions in several African countries, including Kenya (Gifford 2009). Catholic structures helped church leaders coordinate action across dioceses, set clear policies (based on the Pope's early statements), write national-level policies on AIDS, provide funding for program development, and hire staff (through the national-level Catholic secretariats) who could oversee program implementation. To be clear, not every Catholic diocese or parish addressed the disease early or comprehensively, and many Catholics and non-Catholic leaders would argue that the Catholic Church across Africa did not give the disease as much attention as it warranted (Kelly 2007). However, when it did act, this hierarchy facilitated Catholic Church activities. For example, when the Ndola diocese in Zambia developed its successful home-based care programs, the Zambia Episcopal Conference (the overarching body for the country's Catholics) helped other dioceses replicate the program. Exchange of information through the Southern African Catholic Bishops' Conference then made it possible to rapidly copy Zambia's model in other African countries.

Some mainline denominations developed relatively early programs and spoke about the need to address AIDS. For example, the Evangelical Presbyterian Church of Ghana, with a sizeable number of its member churches located in the eastern part of the country where HIV rates are among the highest, agreed at its 1994 national synod meeting to mainstream AIDS intervention into youth programs and other church activities (Interview 29; Evangelical Presbyterian Church of Ghana n.d.). Yet a more common pattern for mainline Protestants was for them to work through national-level ecumenical bodies, since congregational autonomy made early, comprehensive action more difficult for them than for the Catholics. Two examples illustrate. In 2002, the Zambian Episcopal Conference (Catholics), Christian Council of Zambia (mainline Protestants), and Evangelical Fellowship of Zambia (primarily Pentecostals) set up a task force to coordinate church AIDS efforts and communicate with nongovernmental organizations (*Post*, March 17, 2002). In 2000, the Zimbabwe Council of Churches (mainline Protestants) called on the government to suspend the AIDS levy, a tax which was intended to raise funds for AIDS programs, after allegations of corruption in the tax authority emerged (*Financial Gazette [Harare]*, January 21, 2000).

The Compassion Campaign in Ghana illustrates the advantages of the ecumenical structure for relatively early action on AIDS. The stated goal of the Christian Council is to "strengthen the capacity of member churches to contribute to achieveing [*sic*] justice, unity, reconciliation and integrity of creation among the various sectors of Ghanaian society and to provide a forum for joint action on issues of common concern" (Christian Council of Ghana 2008). As Chapter 4 illustrates, the council has a history of political and social involvement. Its leaders, often quoted in the newspapers, are some of the most powerful religious voices in the country (*Ghanaian Times*, November 21, 2008), and its professional staff has linkages to global ecumenical organizations and Western mainline Protestant denominations. This structure enabled churches to undertake a high-level AIDS awareness campaign and to speak with one voice on the disease, particularly when individual congregations or denominations were unlikely to do so. Donors felt relatively confident providing campaign funds to the council because of its long history, well-defined organization, and leadership. The ecumenical nature of the campaign also made it less likely that society could criticize particular denominations or that individual congregations would be put off by a certain pastor's actions on AIDS. As a result, the campaign helped to convince congregations and parishioners to accept that AIDS infects and affects both Christians and non-Christians (Interviews 30, 35, 49, 50).

Churches without hierarchical structures or linkages to ecumenical organizations that were active on AIDS had a more difficult time developing early programs. Without exchange of information, coordination across congregations or denominations, and structures of support, autonomous congregations or individual pastors were less likely to address AIDS. This was particularly true before the new millennium, when many political leaders did not publicly discuss the disease and resources for AIDS programs were limited. More autonomous churches lacked an external impetus (such as the national bishops for Catholics or an ecumenical council for mainline Protestant denominations) that could push congregations or individual pastors to act. Church hierarchy facilitated early actions on AIDS, with the Catholic structure encouraging and sustaining the most comprehensive efforts. Later, though, the relative autonomy found in Pentecostal churches enabled pastors with greater power centralization to respond in creative ways to AIDS. I return to this point below.

Participation in Coalitions

National and global coalitions of non-state actors have played an important role in the fight against AIDS, particularly in ensuring ARV access in Africa (Smith and Siplon 2006; Friedman and Mottiar 2004). Coalitions can increase a church's access to resources, augment its voice in the public realm, and bring energy to advocacy (Interviews 7, 17, 23). Churches may be somewhat advantaged over secular groups in coalition formation, since churches are "present in communities all over the world" (WCC 2001). At the local level, they interact directly with citizens, while globally they may be linked to ecumenical organizations such as the World Council of Churches, the World Pentecostal Fellowship, or the All Africa Conference of Churches. (I devote more attention to global ecumenical relationships in Chapter 5.)

I analyze three variations in such collaboration: (1) coalitions between various churches; (2) coalitions between churches and non-Christian religious groups; (3) and formal and informal cooperation between churches and people living with HIV/AIDS. I then suggest reasons for these coalitions, and more specifically, their implications for inter-religious relations and for participation of people living with HIV/AIDS in church AIDS responses. As the interviewees point out, coalitions are not cost free; they require members to compromise; they necessitate constant communication and sensitivity to others' needs; and they demand time and effort. In Zambia, such challenges included debates about who set priorities for religious coalitions and how those priorities should be communicated (Interviews 10, 17, 20). Similarly, Uganda's Inter-Religious Council faced charges from leaders of African traditional religions that it was exclusionary (Uganda Religious Leaders 2010).

The Expanded Church Response in Zambia illustrates the first pattern. After encouragement from World Vision-Zambia, several pastors, including the leader of the Northmead Assembly of God, formed the group in 2000. It was intended to give churches one focus on the epidemic and to strategically place them for advocacy. The Expanded Church Response represents faith-based organizations on the Zambian National HIV/AIDS/STI/TB Council (NAC), and it was a large catalyst in pastoral opposition to explicit condom advertisements in 2002 (Interviews 7, 8, 9; Expanded Church Response n.d.). Such an inter-church coalition was possible because, as noted previously, churches tend to be relatively conservative on issues such as condom distribution and abstinence education, even churches that stress biblical themes of compassion, love, and the *image deo*. This inter-church coalition also focused on capacity building and accessing resources, not biblical debates. For example, the Expanded Church Response trains church members and leaders to write reports, oversee accounts, and communicate with international partners (Interview 11).

Churches in many countries have worked across religious lines. Catholics, Muslims, and Protestants (primarily Old and New Mission churches) worked together on Ghana's Compassion Campaign; the project also included the secular Ghana AIDS Network. Uganda's Inter-Religious Council brings together the Church of Uganda Anglican, the Orthodox Church, the Seventh Day Adventists, the Roman Catholic Church, and the Uganda Muslim Supreme Council to implement abstinence and marital fidelity workshops and to provide palliative care through its religious members. Begun around 2005, these programs have received support from donors such as USAID (IRCU n.d.) In Zambia, the Catholic Church, mainline Protestants, Pentecostals, and the Expanded Church Response have worked with individuals from the Muslim, Hindu, and Baha'i faith in the Zambia Interfaith Networking

Group on HIV/AIDS (ZINGO). ZINGO began in 1997 when religious leaders met to strategize about ways to "use religion to preserve life." A year later, the group developed a manual, "Treasuring the Gift of Sex," to help religious leaders frame AIDS in the context of frank discussions about sexual relationships. After consultation with UNAIDS, the group decided to scale up its coordination to the national level, and by 2003, ZINGO had formal structures, a written constitution, and official state recognition. Despite their different religious backgrounds, all ZINGO members regard "AIDS as a problem arising from society's inability to holistically address the socio-economic challenges facing humans," and the organization demonstrates solidarity against AIDS among all people of faith (UNAIDS 2008c, 61).

Several factors facilitated these inter-religious coalitions. First, faith leaders recognize that AIDS is a pressing issue that negatively affects society and, as crucial societal actors, religious groups cannot ignore the disease. Second, religious leaders increasingly see a need for a coordinated voice in the AIDS policy realm, because donors demand such representation and because AIDS institutions are growing more complicated and bureaucratic. Churches seek participation in cross-religious groups to facilitate access to power and resources through this institutional mire. Western secular donors also value inter-religious cooperation because it shows tolerance for religious pluralism. (It is notable that donors such as USAID and UNAIDS assisted the Uganda, Ghanaian, and Zambian inter-religious coalitions mentioned above). Additionally, religious actors in these groups have been willing to focus on technical issues, such as capacity building and leadership training, instead of ideological debates. These religious leaders have often agreed to disagree and to let each member organization deal with controversial issues in light of its own religious doctrine (Uganda Religious Leaders 2010; IRCU n.d.). In the case of Uganda, this avoidance of difficult issues may be possible, in part, because one of the most outspoken pastors on sexual morality—Pastor Martin Ssempa—does not participate in the Inter-Religious Council.

The aforementioned coalitions are situated within Christian-majority countries, a fact which allows churches to play a central role in these efforts. This dominance is rooted in colonial history, when churches often acted as arms of the state, particularly in socioeconomic development. Higher levels of education among Christian leaders than among Muslim or African traditional religious leaders also facilitated this privileged position (Morgan 2010; Gifford 1998). Christian and Muslim leaders have sometimes been suspicious of African traditional religions, fearing that syncretism would weaken the faith (Cooper 2006).

In some countries, such concerns have led state officials to exclude leaders of African traditional religions from AIDS resources or to blame these religious groups for violence against people with AIDS (Uganda Religious Leaders 2010).

Because churches in Christian-majority countries have played this prominent role within AIDS institutions, they may have greater access to state and donor resources. Friendships and family relationships forged with state officials through common educational experiences, often in church-related schools, provide these elite linkages that give churches additional leverage in inter-religious coalitions. In a post-September 11 world, Western donors tend to favor Christian over Muslim organizations. For example, over 90 percent of USAID funding for faith-based organizations goes to Christian groups (Patterson 2006, 152). This places Muslim groups working on AIDS in a difficult position; they cannot easily access Western donor funds, but Muslim countries such as Saudi Arabia that have given development monies to African Muslim groups for schools or clinics have had little interest in AIDS (Uganda Religious Leaders 2010). Competition over AIDS resources may lead to suspicion and limited trust between religious groups (IRCU 2010). This tension is set within a context in which roughly one-fourth of Ghanaians and Ugandans viewed religious conflict to be a "very big problem." (Only 7% of Zambians had the same belief.) (Pew Forum 2010) While inter-religious AIDS coalitions did not lead to conflict, they may be perceived by religious minorities as another avenue by which they are excluded from power and representation.

The third type of collaboration is between churches and people living with HIV/AIDS. A major hallmark of the global AIDS movement has been the mobilization of people living with HIV/AIDS. In the West, particularly during the early years of the epidemic, organizations such as the AIDS Coalition to Unleash Power (ACT UP) and Gay Men's Health Crisis helped to forge a common identity among their HIV-positive members and to shape policy outcomes. In so doing, they empowered people living with HIV/AIDS to make autonomous health decisions and to develop distinct forms of political mobilization (Smith and Siplon 2006; Siplon 2010). The incorporation of HIV-positive people into church AIDS responses in Africa has been somewhat different. It has not always been people with the disease who have mobilized, but rather church leaders, pastors, and officers at church-run health centers who have the political and educational skills to mobilize on behalf of those living with HIV/AIDS. While many of these leaders no doubt have been affected by AIDS, they were not necessarily all infected. And for those who were, many did not want to disclose their sero-status, because of the stigma associated with the disease. These dynamics shape church relations with HIV-positive individuals in two ways.

First, churches have often missed opportunities to support people living with HIV/AIDS. In one example, scholars detailed how religious organizations in Tanzania did not provide targeted support programs to help HIV-positive believers (Watt et al. 2009). This silence and inaction deters disclosure, particularly if the religious believer does not need to disclose in order to receive particular benefits such as food or ARVs through any AIDS support group (Burchardt 2010). While many HIV-positive African religious leaders have joined ANERELA+ and some HIV-positive clergy have played public roles in AIDS politics, many churches have not specifically put HIV-positive members in decision-making positions. No interviewee mentioned the crucial ideals of the UNAIDS principle Greater Involvement of People Living with HIV/AIDS. Accepted at the 1994 Paris AIDS Summit by over forty countries, the doctrine emphasizes that others should not represent the interests of people with the disease in program development and implementation or policy decisions (UNAIDS 2010a). As a result of this limited representation, church programs sometimes did not meet the actual needs of people living with HIV/AIDS (Interviews 36, 41), and church leaders sometimes treated those with HIV/AIDS in patronizing ways (Banda 2009).

The second theme is collaboration between churches and secular organizations comprised of people living with HIV/AIDS. Unlike in the United States, where (primarily) gay activists in AIDS organizations were often not also church members, in Africa there often is an overlap in membership between an AIDS group and a religious institution. Despite this fact, large-scale collaboration like that seen between the Treatment Action Campaign and the South African Council of Churches on the issue of universal ARV access has not been replicated in other countries (Friedman and Mottiar 2004). Zambian churches did not work in direct and concrete ways with the Network of Zambian People Living with HIV/AIDS; the same was true of Ghanaian churches and collaboration with the Society for Women Against AIDS in Africa or the National Association of HIV-Positive People (Interviews 19, 28, 39).

Several reasons underlie this pattern of limited collaboration. First, because of stigma, silence, and discrimination in some churches, HIV-positive believers feared disclosure. This situation discouraged joining AIDS groups. The second reason revolves around patriarchy; many churches espouse conservative gender norms that made it "hard to work with churches on gender and AIDS" (Interview 39). Since the majority of members of organizations that represent people living with

HIV/AIDS are women, and gender vulnerability has become a central issue that these AIDS organizations address, patriarchy in the church is problematic for dialogue (Banda 2009). Third, some church leaders thought that these groups often unfairly blamed the church for the disease's stigma, a fact which made churches defensive and hesitant to collaborate (Interview 25). Additionally, groups that represented people living with HIV/AIDS were often organizationally weak, a fact that limited their ability to build coalitions (Interview 34; Banda 2009). One individual involved with AIDS policy-making in Ghana explained:

> [Groups that represent people with HIV/AIDS] are not strong enough. This is because of their small size, and their leadership is not strong. They lack technical knowledge.... They could do so much more if they came together in coalitions. ... Civil society is instrumental for change, but they need coalitions or networks to make change. [They lack] the capacity to cooperate or to build ties across different groups. (Interview 27)

Overall, any type of collaboration (inter-church, inter-religious, or church-secular AIDS group) did not seem to determine the timing or breadth of church AIDS efforts. Early Catholic action was not rooted in coalitions. In fact, many church-related coalitions on AIDS did not form until the late-1990s, when the Catholics had already begun many programs.[23] Even in the case of Ghana's Compassion Campaign, the inter-religious coalition began to dissipate after the campaign ended and donor interest in the country's epidemic dwindled. For churches with more recent AIDS efforts, coalitions do not appear to have caused these actions. Instead, they seem to have reinforced churches' AIDS activities, particularly the more broadly-focused ones. For example, the Expanded Church Response in Zambia receives Global Fund money, works with multinational nongovernmental organizations such as World Vision and Family Health International, and gets support from USAID (PEPFAR 2007; Interview 8). These resources are then channeled to member churches. For the Northmead Assembly of God, these connections helped to solidify the church's own programs and to amplify the pastor's voice in policy-making on AIDS. Similarly, UNAIDS (2008c) reports that inter-church and inter-religious coalitions are one of the most successful aspects of Zambia's AIDS efforts. Overall, Zambian interviewees viewed coalitions positively (Interviews 14, 16, 23, 25), with one respondent explaining that the only problem with them is that there "just aren't enough of them" (Interview 23). But, the limited incorporation of people living with HIV/AIDS into the church power structures that designed AIDS responses (particularly the more narrowly focused programs) presents a challenge to the representation and inclusivity of church AIDS efforts. Greater inclusion of people living with HIV/AIDS into decision making has the potential to increase the effectiveness and legitimacy of church AIDS responses.

In sum, church hierarchy, particularly as seen in the Catholic Church, made it more likely that churches would act before 2001 to combat AIDS. Catholic hierarchy probably also made it more likely such efforts would incorporate a variety of responses including care, stigma reduction, prevention, and support. In the case of Protestants, the ecumenical council structures found in most countries helped facilitate church collaboration on AIDS awareness, as was evident in Ghana's Compassion Campaign. Hierarchy helped churches implement AIDS programs, when they might not have done so in the pre-2001 environment because the disease was not on the political agenda. On the other hand, when the pandemic became a priority, church hierarchy seemed to matter less for urging church actions. As the next section argues, the relatively recent emergence of Pentecostal pastors with an AIDS agenda is not solely a result of Pentecostal organizational structures but also of charismatic and visionary leaders. Coalitions, often under-developed and sometimes mired in unequal power relations, may reinforce church power on AIDS, but because these forms of collaboration were relatively recent constructions and because they often did not incorporate people living with HIV/AIDS, they did not influence the timing or scope of church AIDS activities.

Pastoral Leadership

Pastors hold powerful positions in African society because of the centrality of religion on the continent. Table 3.1 illustrates the percentage of survey respondents in select Christian-majority countries who said that religion was "somewhat or very important" in their lives (Little and Logan 2008, 30).[24] The second column gives the percentage of respondents who self-identify as a leader or member of a religious organization. Although not all of these individuals are active members (in some countries 40 to 50% say they are inactive), these numbers are noticeably greater than the percentage of respondents who report membership in a voluntary or community organization (see the table's third column). Even in countries with relatively low participation in religious organizations (e.g., Cape Verde and Lesotho), involvement in religious organizations is at least 10 percent higher than it is in secular organizations. In most countries, the gap is over 30 percentage points.

Country[1]	Religion is somewhat or very important (%)	Leader or member of religious group (%)	Leader or member of voluntary or community organization (%)
Botswana	79	67	21
Burundi	93	77	47
Cape Verde	78	41	25
Ghana	93	87	45
Kenya	95	88	55
Lesotho	95	56	43
Malawi	94	88	32
Namibia	92	74	27
South Africa	80	62	29
Tanzania	94	77	42
Uganda	94	73	44

Source: Afrobarometer 2009, 30

[1] *For the 2009 report, Afrobarometer conducted surveys in eighteen countries. The eleven listed have a Christian majority. The other countries were Benin, Liberia, Madagascar, Mali, Mozambique, Nigeria, and Senegal.*

The centrality of religion, as well as the weakness of other civil society organizations, explains why many Africans turn to religious leaders when they have problems. A 2006 Gallup survey conducted in nineteen African countries found that religious organizations are the most trusted institutions on the continent, with 76 percent of respondents having confidence in them (Gallup News Service 2007). In 2009, the Afrobarometer survey found that 40 percent of respondents in eighteen surveyed countries had contacted a religious leader about a problem at least once during the last year. In contrast, 24 percent had contacted a traditional leader and 27 percent had contacted a local government official (Afrobarometer 2009, 11). In Zambia, a country with a large Christian majority (see Table 1.1), 56 percent of respondents in 2005 claimed to have seen a religious leader at least once during the last year (Afrobarometer 2005). Michael Bratton and Wonbin Cho (2006, 38) write, "Even after 50 years of African independence, organized religion looms much larger in the life [*sic*] of ordinary Africans than does the apparatus of the state." Secular and religious respondents echoed the point that religious leaders are influential and respected figures (Interviews 16, 25, 27, 34).

African Christians rely on pastors because of these leaders' organizational, speaking, and mobilizing skills, and their perceived trustworthiness. In many communities, pastors are the most, or the only, educated citizens (Green 2003). As community leaders, they have connections to other civil society groups, state officials, and/or local elites. And as intermediaries between the spiritual and physical worlds, pastors are perceived to have unique powers such as the gifts of healing, prophecy, speaking in tongues, and/or spiritual intercession. Because spiritual power is as real in Africa as physical power, and because few (if any) other community members can claim such spiritual linkages, pastors have a unique form of legitimacy (Meyer 2004; Ellis and ter Haar 1998). Because pastors are people "chosen by God" with "one hand in the spiritual world," church members may believe these leaders are above the influence of state patronage or the temptation to misuse church funding (Christiansen 2009; Ellis and ter Haar 1998, 191-192; FBO Roundtable 2009). Even though such assumptions about accountability can be challenged, they help increase the influence of pastors in public debates.

Pastoral leadership can shape church AIDS efforts in several ways. First, some pastors have ignored the disease, propagated the stigma against AIDS, or spread inaccurate information about the epidemic. In so doing, they contribute to the do-nothing church reaction. One church AIDS worker explained that without the pastor's encouragement, church members will not initiate programs on AIDS (Interview 36). Another activist remarked: “They [pastors] can destroy all our work on treatment education or stigma reduction in a one hour sermon, because people listen to them” (Banda 2009). Negative pastoral reactions to AIDS may result from biblical perspectives (as outlined earlier), but they also may reflect the fact that pastors sometimes lack accurate information about the disease. Swaziland’s National Emergency Response Committee on HIV/AIDS found that even pastors on the committee disseminated incorrect information about AIDS (*UN Integrated Regional Information Network*, July 19, 2007). A Ghanaian pastor explained how this situation can occur:

> Apart from the medical professionals and health workers, church workers are not trained on AIDS. They want to work on the issue because it affects the church and its people. … But people need training to be able to carry on with an issue, so that it becomes their own issue. … Pastors are trained [for] preaching and teaching. Then you add AIDS onto this situation, and that makes it hard without support (Interview 30).

The interviewee’s larger point was that pastors need continued education to adequately lead their churches’ AIDS responses.

Second, some pastors have urged their churches to respond to the epidemic through spiritual healing. Healing has always been a crucial component of Pentecostalism, but the emergence of “health and wealth” churches at roughly the same time that the number of AIDS cases in Africa exploded has increased the appeal of this message. The adoption of neoliberal economic policies in the 1980s and 1990s that contributed to unprecedented economic challenges has further heightened the appeal of the health and wealth emphasis (Dilger 2007, 66; Gifford 1998; Sackey 2006). Pentecostal churches with this emphasis stress that salvation from evil includes relief from distress, poverty, and disease. Pastors are central in these healing ministries, because they are assumed to be directly linked to God. Additionally, their sometimes ostentatious lifestyles fuel the belief that God gives material blessings to those who serve him. Thus, some pastors may lead churches to adopt the narrow, spiritual healing approach to AIDS.

Third, pastors may create symbolic and rhetorical contexts in which AIDS can either be addressed or denied. Robin Root (2009) describes how the pastor of a Swazi church used the language and imagery of personhood to foster a belief in the dignity of all people, including those living with HIV/AIDS. The pastor’s actions, which included personally washing the feet of church home-based care workers, powerfully symbolized themes of Christian service and humility, particularly since social hierarchies in Africa can be rigid and pastors are viewed to be high in social status. Using rhetoric about courage, the pastor created an environment in which parishioners felt they could disclose their HIV status. In another example, the Niassa Diocese of Mozambique's Anglican Church named its teams of home-based care givers *equipas de vida* (or, teams of life). This language emphasized both the biblical reference to Jesus Christ as the means to eternal life and demonstrated the possibility of a full life for people living with HIV/AIDS (Vander Meulen 2010).[25]

Fourth, pastors have acted as entrepreneurs or visionaries who have capitalized on increased global and national interest in AIDS in the new millennium to develop both narrow and broad efforts. As Bishop Joshua Banda and Pastor Martin Ssempa illustrate, many of these individuals serve urban Pentecostal churches. While a hallmark of Pentecostalism has always been dynamic preaching and healing, pastors now augment that skill with increased educational training, greater professionalism, savvy political skills, and links to Western churches. Increased power centralization around the pastor means that the pastor's personality and priorities may have a high degree of influence on church programs.

In some ways, these Pentecostal pastors resemble the model of personal rule seen in African politics (Rosberg and Jackson 1982). As charismatic leaders, they use personal networks to allocate resources, make decisions, and urge action to fulfill their visions. While they may make public pronouncements (through sermons or media statements) to set agendas, they also utilize private conversations and meetings with small groups of parishioners to motivate action. These behind-the-scenes activities are particularly important in large churches, because they get congregants incorporated into church life. Personal relations forged in these groups foster accountability among members and may be more crucial than prayer or attendance at religious services for motivating believers to participate in voluntary service to others (Adamczyk 2010). The Watoto church in Kampala (formerly the Kampala Pentecostal Church) provides an example. As an urban, mega-church with over two thousand worshippers, the church has the potential to foster distance among parishioners and between its leaders and followers. During the church's three Sunday services that are held in a former theater, the pastor stands on a large stage under bright lights with a huge choir behind him. Yet, church members have mobilized on AIDS through the church's cell groups, which provide teams for care and support to congregants and neighbors with AIDS. Church pastors helped create this environment of belonging by urging small group formation and participation.[26]

Additionally, pastors' personal ties to external actors or the state may help to bring material benefits to their organizations (Patterson 1998; Fatton 1995; Chabal and Daloz 1999). Pastors "accumulate resources to operate neo-patrimonial systems of church governance" (Maxwell 2000, 253). Believers define "good pastors" not only in terms of preaching or teaching, but also in light of the traditional belief that leaders (in this case, pastors) are expected to care about and help provide for the material needs of their followers. Such social obligations, or what Goran Hyden terms the "economy of affection," have not disappeared with the emergence of liberal economies or democratic transitions; if anything, many religious followers are disillusioned with the false promises of modernity, democratization, and neoliberalism (Hyden 1980; Scott 1976; Haynes 2009). Some of these pastors have been accused of using their positions and ministries to benefit themselves personally instead of their unemployed, impoverished, and hungry followers (Kalu 2008, 140-146). In some cases, such accusations are accurate. But the material ostentation displayed by some pastors is situated within the African social context in which clients expect patrons to demonstrate power and authority through outward signs such as dress, cars, and houses. A patron's power also is defined by the size of his following (Chabal and Daloz 1999). Religious patrons compete for believers, and, as David Maxwell (2000, 250) found, Pentecostal churches in Zimbabwe are "subject to intense struggles for resources, power and clients."

Another element of personal rule is the use of symbols to increase a leader's power (Moss 2007, 37). To propagate this symbolic legitimacy, some Pentecostal pastors have taken the titles of "bishop," "apostle," or "prophet," words that link them to the African founders of the Old Independent Churches or that signify God's choice of these individuals for ministry (Kalu 2008). These pastors often recount their own spiritual conversion experiences (being "born again") and their material successes, stories which demonstrate God's power over evil and his ability to bring victory and prosperity. To reach local and global audiences, Pentecostal pastors adeptly use the tools of globalization, such as cell phones, websites, blogs, emailed newsletters, international speaking engagements, and cable television shows. My point is not to criticize Pentecostal pastors as neopatrimonial leaders. Instead, I wish to situate them in a larger social context in which leaders (religious, secular, state, and non-state) are expected to use their skills, connections, and symbolic power to provide material help to their followers. The relatively autonomous structure of many Pentecostal churches enables pastors to use these tools to creatively define their ministries, including on AIDS.

To be clear, pastoral leadership is important in all churches, but as the previous section argued, there is more freedom for pastors to act in Pentecostal churches because of the churches' autonomous structures and centralization of power. These autonomous structures provide space in which pastors can use their charisma, visions for programs, prior experiences, and networks to shape AIDS responses. While pastors in mainline Protestant or Catholic churches may possess similar skills, Pentecostal pastors often have more opportunity to capitalize on those skills, as the following examples of Bishop Joshua Banda at the Northmead Assembly of God in Lusaka and Pastor Martin Ssempa at the Makerere Community Church in Kampala illustrate. I analyze how these leaders' personal characteristics led to their churches' participation in AIDS activities.

The first noticeable aspect of these two pastors' leadership is the way they capitalize on their personal stories to legitimate their activities. In doing so, their personal stories echo some of the above-mentioned aspects of Pentecostal leadership. At age fourteen, Banda experienced a spiritual rebirth that led him to ministry when he turned eighteen. Over the years, he has served as the secretary for the Southern Africa Assemblies of God Association (2003-2007) and the principal of the Trans-Africa Theological College in Kitwe, Zambia (1990-1995). He has studied theology in the United States, and as of 2010 Banda was conducting research on community-based HIV prevention for his dissertation from the Centre for Mission Studies at Oxford University. Even though Banda and the Northmead Assembly of God strongly support HIV prevention through abstinence and fidelity programs, the bishop's experiences have propelled a comprehensive approach to AIDS. With larger links to the Assemblies of God in Africa and as the former head of a center of theological education, he no doubt has encountered a wide variety of challenges that churches have faced that relate to care, support, treatment, stigma reduction, and prevention.

Similarly, Ssempa uses his own personal story to ground his church's narrow prevention efforts. In video clips on his website, he recounts how as a teen, he was "Mr. Break Dance of East Africa," with girlfriends and a fast lifestyle. When a girlfriend got pregnant and his brother and sister-in-law died of AIDS in the early 1990s, he began to re-evaluate his life. He describes how his brother's HIV infection resulted from "sex outside of marriage," a fact that instilled fear in the pastor and caused him to change his sexual behavior (Ssempa 2009). His professional experience also helps legitimate his AIDS activities. Trained in sociology at Makerere University and biblical counseling in Philadelphia, Ssempa worked as an AIDS case manager in the United States before returning to Uganda and founding the Makerere Church (*Monitor*, March 10, 2004). According to his website, he has "over twenty years of experience" with AIDS, although it is unclear if all this experience was in Uganda (Ssempa 2009).

Second, these pastors have developed AIDS programs that resonate with their church congregants; they astutely understand their own church audiences. Banda's congregation is relatively well educated, older, and middle class. While they are concerned about youth sexual activity, they are also concerned about the effects of AIDS on the community (Interview 7). In contrast, Ssempa's church audience is primarily college students who, living on a college campus and experiencing youthful sexual desires, face the "temptation" of premarital sex. Because of their stage in life, many are also concerned about finding a marriage partner and eventually, having a family. Hence, Ssempa's abstinence and fidelity messages resonate, particularly for some youth who may be more likely than adults to see the world in terms of moral dichotomies. For Ssempa, a key aspect of his AIDS prevention programs is to make young people fear AIDS: "Fear based messages work" (Ssempa 2009).

Alessandro Gusman (2009) points to an additional reason why these youth-focused messages work in the Ugandan context: they juxtapose the alleged moral behavior of today's youth with the alleged immorality of past generations. For many of these young born-again Christians, it was the corruption, misuse of power, and debauchery of their parents' generation (and the mission churches that their parents attended) that facilitated a context in which HIV infections could spread rapidly. Uganda's poverty and high youth unemployment fuels the generational conflict embedded in such messages.

Because many African churches have developed links to international faith-based organizations and Western churches, each of these pastors has a larger audience beyond the immediate congregation. Banda's broader audience includes both international donors and the Pentecostal community in southern Africa. For the first group, he has sought to gain greater empirical support for the efficacy of his churches' efforts. Arguing that faith-based organizations can be "weak in documentation," the bishop asserts that his dissertation research on faith-based abstinence and fidelity programs can help provide concrete evidence to assist church advocacy for HIV prevention programs (UNAIDS 2008c; FBO Roundtable 2009). The bishop appears to be responding to calls from donors for "evidence-based" solutions to AIDS

(UNAIDS 2007; Interview 7). For the second group, his broad approach to AIDS enables him to work with a variety of church leaders in organizations such as the Expanded Church Response.

Ssempa's broader audience includes conservative Ugandans and some conservative American evangelical churches. His anti-homosexual statements and activities (detailed more in Chapter 5) resonate with Ugandans from a variety of religious backgrounds. They have supported his positions, although rarely in the bold language he has used (Interview 61; Uganda Religious Leaders 2010). In informal discussions with educated and somewhat progressive Ugandans, I was often struck by their anti-homosexual sentiments and their doubt that homosexuals really exist in Uganda.[27] These sentiments also find support among many American evangelicals, who along with many African Christians and Muslims fear a global gay rights movement (Massad 2002; Interview 61).

Each pastor has developed a style for delivering AIDS messages that resonates with his local and global audiences. Banda's messages are more formal, and his emphasis on education and evidence fits within his congregation. His sermons are well-developed and his Bible study notes, thorough (Northmead Assembly of God 2009). In contrast, Ssempa is more informal with the students. In his sermons and on his website, he dispenses valuable life advice to inexperienced youth, just as a father would. Unlike pastors in some of the larger churches, Ssempa does not preach from a high stage, wear vestments, use sophisticated media images, or create physical distance between his followers and himself. The church meets in a large classroom at Makerere University's School of Veterinary Science, and worshippers sit at wooden school desks. He uses examples that students understand from popular culture. His emphasis on marital fidelity and traditional family are symbolized through his own children's participation in worship songs and dances and through references to his wife in sermons (Epstein 2005; Ssempa 2009).[28]

To reach their broader audiences, both pastors have developed media outlets and imagery. Banda has a weekly television program that is broadcast throughout southern Africa, and Ssempa has a television program he has hosted for many years. Unlike the bishop, who uses media appearances in the conventional media (e.g., newspaper interviews) or his television show to convey his points, Ssempa stages colorful media events. As mentioned in Chapter 2, he has publicly burned condoms in protests, organized abstinence rallies, and, as Chapter 5 illustrates, he has used what some activists consider to be hateful language about sex workers and homosexuals (Human Rights

Watch 2007). During a 2010 worship service, he encouraged congregants to wear t-shirts with "Africa United Against Sodomy" when they gathered to watch the World Cup final match later that evening. A church member modeled the t-shirt, which was bright yellow and seemed to be a play on the MTN cell-phone advertisements found throughout Africa. These billboards showed African soccer players standing proudly and wearing yellow shirts that read "Africa United." After the church service, Ssempa and other church leaders wore the t-shirts during a national television program when they defended their position on homosexuality.[29] These actions may appeal to his student followers, whose energy and idealism can be capitalized on and who are potentially more likely to appreciate media images than their elders. They also garner national and international media coverage, as evidenced by the large number of blog posts, YouTube cites, and Ugandan and international news articles about him.[30]

A third aspect of these pastors' leadership is their ability to forge and capitalize on global relationships. Banda's experiences in southern African church leadership and studying in the United States and United Kingdom enabled him to build relationships with international faith-based organizations, Western churches, and Pentecostals throughout southern Africa (Northmead Assembly of God 2009).[31] When Western governments and faith-based organizations turned their attention to AIDS, Banda was able to capitalize on such linkages to access donor funding for the Northmead Church and the Expanded Church Response (Gill 2006, 128-130).

Ssempa's activities, as well as his work with First Lady Janet Museveni, a born-again Christian who is closely involved in Uganda's AIDS policy-making, helped him forge ties to donors and American evangelical churches. An anecdote from a 2010 Sunday service illustrates: two young men from an American church who had volunteered with the Ugandan church shared their religious testimony. They concluded with words of encouragement, which highlighted the relationship between the American and Ugandan congregations; they wanted parishioners to know that the American congregation prayed continuously for the Ugandan church and that it treasured their relationship.[32] Such ties have been important for AIDS policies, particularly since American evangelical churches mobilized to pressure former President George W. Bush and a Republican-dominated Congress to pass the PEPFAR legislation in 2003.

There seemed to be a reciprocal relationship between Ssempa's ties to American evangelical churches and his emphasis on abstinence and fidelity in HIV prevention. American attention both influences and is influenced by the pastor's activities. Before American churches became interested in AIDS in Africa, the Makerere Church had some AIDS activities. This fact urged American church leaders and more conservative policy makers to incorporate Ssempa's perspectives and invite him to testify about abstinence programs before the US House of Representatives Committee on International Relations, which was then chaired by Illinois Republican Henry Hyde (Ssempa 2005). On the flip side, once there was greater attention to AIDS among American churches and PEPFAR had been passed, some analysts assert Ssempa's anti-condom statements became louder and more frequent (Blumenthal 2009). This increased activity may have further heightened his popularity with some American evangelical leaders. In 2005, Pastor Rick Warren invited Ssempa to speak at an international AIDS conference he organized at his Saddleback Church in California (Ssempa 2009; Morgan 2005). Since then, Warren broke ties with the Ugandan pastor and publicly denounced his anti-homosexual rhetoric in 2009 (*Newsweek*, December 21, 2009). It would be simplistic, however, to assert that religious leaders such as Ssempa or Banda became concerned with AIDS solely because of American interest and funding.

Finally, as patrons who wield power and influence, use their public persona to set agendas, and forge networks to access resources, both pastors are not without domestic and international criticism. In the case of Banda, Zambian interviewees asserted that as a "prominent person" the bishop did not do the difficult work of program development and implementation (Interviews 10, 20). Yet, such criticisms reinforce the point that such pastors act as big men who provide an entrepreneurial vision and then direct others to do the work to fulfill the vision. Criticism of Ssempa focuses on his positions on issues and the dramatic methods he uses to mobilize support for those messages (Interview 61). Yet, it is helpful to remember that the pastor has been able to take these positions and use such strategies because he has a great deal of autonomy in church decision making; he founded the congregation and it appears that he makes many of its decisions (*Monitor*, March 10, 2004).

This section has argued that pastoral leadership can determine how churches respond to AIDS. While the role of church leaders is particularly heightened in the larger Pentecostal churches, pastors are highly influential in all denominations. It is hard to dissect the role of organizational structures from leadership qualities, although the charisma, skills, and experiences of Banda and Ssempa demonstrate that leadership attributes cannot be discounted. Power centralization in pastors who adeptly use the media to mobilize followers and to forge domestic and international connections enables these leaders to be an important variable in church responses. As the next chapter illustrates, some of these pastors have become more involved in state policy-making on AIDS.

Conclusion

This chapter has focused on three types of resources to explain the scope and timing of church actions: biblical frameworks for understanding AIDS, church structures and coalitions, and pastoral leadership. It finds that the biblical themes of compassion and love for all people encouraged early, comprehensive AIDS activities. The focus on God's power—to punish or to heal—has led some churches to ignore the disease, while others focus on spiritual healing. Even though biblical principles of sexual morality have pushed the vast majority of churches to emphasize abstinence and fidelity, churches with a more recent, narrow focus emphasize these ideas and oppose condoms in HIV prevention. Churches that acted early, such as the Catholics and some mainline Protestants, tended to be part of larger hierarchical structures or national ecumenical councils. Coalitions played a minimal role in urging early efforts to fight the disease, but they helped to reinforce and expand later church actions. Some Pentecostal leaders have taken on a new importance in more recent AIDS efforts, particularly because their access to media outlets and relative autonomy in church decision making have empowered them to develop new initiatives and access external resources.

Three implications emerge from the chapter's findings. First, biblical principles—or the frameworks that shape what members and leaders believe—have a considerable impact on church AIDS responses. The civil society literature devotes little attention to ideas as drivers of institutional outcomes, although the social movement literature has paid more attention to such questions in its examination of collective identity (Stryker, Owens, and White 2000). Of course, not all members of any civil society group or broader social movement share the same perspective on problems, and even if they do, they may not live up to the high ideals they espouse. But, beliefs cannot be dismissed in any analysis of religion and politics in Africa. Second, the findings raise questions about the role of Africa's mainline Protestant churches on AIDS and more broadly, African social change. Some of these churches, such as the Presbyterians, Lutherans, and Methodists, lack an overall hierarchy to push AIDS activities from the top, but they also lack congregational autonomy that permits "go-it-alone" pastors with a vision for AIDS programs to act. While some of these churches have acted on AIDS, sometimes on their own, but more often with support from national and global ecumenical councils, their organizational structure can present a challenge for these churches' ability to sustain long-term AIDS responses. Finally, in churches where pastors have been central to AIDS programs, what might happen if these pastors' priorities change? The crucial role of pastors in such efforts raises questions about the long-term sustainability and accountability of these churches' responses in the fight against HIV and AIDS.

---

[1] Pastoral leadership refers to any clergy member, including Catholic priests.

[2] Several participants at the 2009 meeting of the International Research Network on Religion and AIDS in Africa pointed to the contrasting ways that churches have used the Hebrew Bible and New Testament to motivate AIDS responses. Author observations, Lusaka, Zambia, April 15-17, 2009.

[3] The term Hebrew Bible has become the more accepted reference for the thirty-nine books that are found in both the Jewish canon (*Tanakh*) and the Protestant canon. (Roman Catholic and Eastern Orthodox churches include additional writings.) It replaces the term Old Testament, which was problematic because Christians did not agree on which books were included in the Old Testament and because its usage implied that all the stories in the Bible (in both Old and New Testaments) were uniquely Christian. The Hebrew Bible contains the creation story, the history of the ancient Israelites (who lived before Christianity emerged), the warnings of the prophets, and the prophecy of the Messiah's coming. The Christian New Testament (twenty-seven books) highlights the birth, ministry, crucifixion, and resurrection of God's son Jesus Christ, the spread of Christianity by Christ's disciples, and the founding of the early church.

[4] I use male pronouns to refer to God out of conventionality, not because I think God has a specific gender.

[5] This point about the lack of resources for pastors and seminaries was often repeated at the Network for African Congregational Theology Conference on AIDS, Poverty, and the Church which I attended in Lusaka, Zambia, August 4-11, 2007.

[6] Examples of such texts include Exodus 20:14, Leviticus 18:22, Leviticus 20:10-13, Romans 1:26-27, and Matthew 5:27-28. Genesis 18 and 19 report that God destroys Sodom and Gomorrah because the people had turned against God's ways, specifically by committing adultery and homosexual acts.

[7] See the story of Cain and Abel in Genesis 4. Ostracizing, shunning, and ignoring also illustrate a congregation's fear of HIV and AIDS or the concern that the alleged sins of the HIV-positive member will damage the congregation's reputation.

[8] See Genesis 2:18-24, Genesis 24:58-60, Malachi 2:14, and Matthew 19:6.

[9]See Matthew 5:32, Romans 7:2-3, and Hebrews 13:4.

[10] During the four months of church services I attended in Ghana, I never heard discussion about marital fidelity. The issue of multiple partners came up indirectly when a female elder in a middle-class, interdenominational church announced a church-sponsored health program on cosmetics. She invited the men to attend the program, so they would "know about cosmetics to buy for their wives or …" Although she did not say mistress (and did not mean to imply it), everyone in the congregation snickered, as if they knew that many men had girlfriends (author observation, Accra, November 16, 2008). An interviewee confirmed my interpretation of the event (Interview 43).

[11] For an example of this potentially stigmatizing rhetoric, Krakauer and Newbery (2007, 33) cite a South African Zionist pastor: "If you get killed by AIDS, it is you who expose yourself to it… Maybe it is only you who is affected, but you will end up destroying the whole community."

[12] See Genesis 17:15-21, 2 Kings 5:1-4, and Matthew 4:23.

[13] Belief in witches is widespread among all Africans, including Christians. In the documentary *Witches in Exile*, John Kirby, an expert on religion at the Tamale Institute for Cross Cultural Study in Ghana, asserts that 101 percent of Ghanaians believe in witches (Berg 2005). Helen Epstein describes how Pastor Ssempa told her about the witches that meet under Lake Victoria (quoted in Blumenthal 2009; see also Bornstein 2005, 145-167).

[14] The negative publicity these healing camps have received has caused some camps to "dump" dying AIDS patients at hospitals, after these individuals have no chance for recovery (Interview 47). An informal conversation with a Ghanaian anthropologist on April 15, 2009 echoed these points.

[15] See Matthew 25:31-46.

[16] See Luke 10:25-35.

[17] See Luke 18:35-42, Matthew 9:9-12, Luke 5:12-15, and Luke 8:43-48.

[18] See John 8:1-11.

[19] This observation was conveyed to me by an anthropologist doing field work with faith-based organizations in rural Uganda. Email correspondence with author, June 26, 2009.

[20] For example, a 2005 World Council of Churches report explains: "Sexuality should not be viewed as a taboo topic and open discussion about sexual issues needs to be encouraged. Churches need to speak about relationships, the positive aspects of sexuality as well as being open to discussing sexual health issues. The extent of the HIV pandemic is such that we need to overcome shyness in relation to sexuality and start talking about it in a constructive way." (WCC 2005b; see also Ecumenical Advocacy Alliance n.d.)

[21] After hearing the phrase so often, I finally asked one interviewee who works on HIV/AIDS education in several countries if the lack of capacity had become "just an excuse" for some churches to not do more to address the disease. The individual agreed that while the phrase had become a buzzword, it was also true that some churches did lack capacity to do AIDS work. Informal conversation with ecumenical AIDS educator, Lusaka, Zambia, April 16, 2009.

[22] There is variety in autonomy even within specific denominations. For example, in the Assemblies of God some congregations have full autonomy from a General Council, while others have not yet developed to the point where they are self-governing and self-financing (World Assemblies of God

Fellowship 2009). The Pew Forum provides information on these denominations and Pentecostalism in general (see http://pewforum.org/docs/?DocID=140#advocacy).

[23] Many secular AIDS organizations and coalitions also did not start until the mid-1990s. For example, the Ghana HIV/AIDS Network formed in 1996, South Africa's Treatment Action Campaign began in 1998, South Africa's National Association of People with AIDS formed in 1994, and the Botswana Network of People Living with HIV/AIDS started in 2000 (Patterson 2006, 97-98; see also http://www.bonepwa.botsnet.co.bw).

[24] In contrast, in a 2002 survey, 59 percent of Americans and 30 percent of Canadians said religion was very important in their lives (Pew Global Attitudes Project 2002).

[25] See John 14: 6.

[26] I am grateful to Alessandro Gusman for sharing this point about cell groups and pastoral leadership in the Watoto Church. Author observations, Watoto Church, Kampala, Uganda, July 4, 2010. More information is available at http://www.watotochurch.com.

[27] Informal conversations between author and two Ugandan graduate students, Kampala, Uganda, July 1, 2010 and July 11, 2010.

[28]In one example, he used Ghana's loss in the World Cup as an analogy for the need for Christian discipline. Author observations, Makerere Community Church, Kampala, Uganda, July 11, 2010.

[29] Author observations, Makerere Community Church, Kampala, Uganda, July 11, 2010.

[30] In a quick Google search on July 20, 2010, there were over 100,000 hits with references to Ssempa.

[31] The church's website reports that the bishop is a "highly sought after international conference speaker" (Northmead Assembly of God 2009).

[32] Author observations, Makerere Community Church, Kampala, Uganda, July 11, 2010. The presence of American evangelical church members at Ugandan Pentecostal churches is not unusual, particularly during the summer months when American church members participate in short-term mission experiences abroad. During the July 4, 2010 Watoto church service I observed, the pastor introduced three different groups from the United States.

4

Power and Subversion in Church-State Relations

> "'Big Men' Accused: Grave Looting for Human Parts; Bones Used in Rituals for Political Power" (front page headline of *Ghanaian Times,* October 27, 2008)

> Zimbabwean state officials urged the churches to "continue to work closely with the Government in poverty alleviation… and the fight against HIV/AIDS." (*Herald*, August 23, 2007)

> "There appear [in the church's high leadership] those people who use their voice and have political ambitions. We often say that who [claims to] speak for our denomination or congregation is aspiring to be the next president of the country." (Interview 10)

As these quotations demonstrate, the relationship between politics and religion is fluid in Africa. While most African constitutions officially establish secular governments, the state and church often seem to overlap and influence each other. Politicians seek spiritual protection in Ghana; political leaders in Zimbabwe call on churches to cooperate with the state on AIDS; and Zambian church leaders are perceived to use their positions in religious institutions as stepping stones toward a political career.

Such interactions occur in a political environment of weak state capacity and limited state legitimacy. After roughly fifty years of independence, the African state still cannot adequately provide for the health, education, security, and livelihood of most citizens. Centralization of power in the executive and neopatrimonial politics based on personal networks rather than legal-rational norms contribute to the lack of accountability and weakness in the African state (van de Walle 2001; Moss 2007). Over two decades of neoliberal economic reforms have eroded state capacity; underpaid and overworked civil servants have been demoralized, drawn to the burgeoning sector of nongovernmental organizations, or driven to emigrate to the West (van de Walle 2001; Englebert 2000; Manuh 2005). As a result, Africans show relatively low levels of confidence in state officials and institutions (Little and Logan 2008). State weakness has greatly affected AIDS efforts, as the shortage of doctors, lab technicians, and nurses for ARV treatment programs illustrates (*Boston Globe,* August 21, 2006; Mills et al. 2008).

In this context, religion may be viewed as a threat to the state. Churches possess "moral extraterritoriality" because they may serve as an arena of free thought, speech, and action away from state control (Weigel 1992, 151). By sponsoring development projects such as orphan feeding programs or neighborhood micro-finance efforts, religious institutions fill a void in state services. While service provision helps attract church members, particularly in the newer Pentecostal churches (Jenkins 2007), it also implicitly (and sometimes explicitly) highlights the inability or unwillingness of the state to meet its obligations to citizens. As a result, citizens may see no need to give loyalty to the state (Bates 2008; Patterson 1999). And, as one interviewee pointed out, what is the meaning of citizen rights and responsibilities when the state has been absent in people's lives for more than a generation? (Interview 61) In a direct challenge to state authority, some church leaders have linked poor governance to weak or corrupt state efforts on social service provision. For example, Reverend Henry Orombi, the Archbishop of the Church of Uganda, complained that political incompetence and poor visionary leadership led the Ministry of Health to mismanage Global Fund grants in 2005 (*Monitor*, September 26, 2005).

Churches also can challenge the state simply because of their perceived link to the spiritual world. Stephen Ellis and Gerrie ter Haar (2004, 8) explain, "Politicians seek power. In African societies, power is widely thought to originate in the spirit world." As the aforementioned newspaper headline on the alleged grave robbing by Ghanaian candidates illustrates, politicians may try to use the spirit realm to advance their careers or to protect themselves from their opponents' evil intentions. Politicians such as former Kenyan president Daniel arap Moi and Ghanaian coup-maker Colonel Acheampong consulted exorcists, Pentecostal pastors, and spiritualists when they desired protection from their enemies (Ellis and ter Haar 1998; Pobee 1991). In 2003, the financially bankrupt Ghana Airways held an all-night prayer vigil in hopes of resurrecting the company, which had been destroyed by mismanagement and corruption (Asamoah-Gyadu 2005a).

This chapter examines church-state dynamics to elucidate why some churches have adopted particular approaches to AIDS. While I pay particular attention to churches that have engaged in political advocacy, I recognize that responses to the disease are often inter-related and advocacy is rarely a church's sole activity. I divide the chapter into three main parts. In the first, I dissect four aspects of the church-state relationship and analyze their effects on church AIDS actions: (1) past church political involvement, particularly in Africa's democratic transitions of the early 1990s; (2) a church's political theology, or its doctrine of political involvement; (3) church-state cooperation in health care provision; (4) church representation on the Global Fund-mandated Country Coordinating Mechanisms (CCM). In the second part, I question how the larger political and religious environment in which churches operate may condition their AIDS actions. This section looks at the assumed political opportunities that occurred with democratization after 1990. Because this pluralism also created opportunities for new church formation, I investigate the larger religious environment. Since the book's focus is church actions to address AIDS, I devote most attention to the first and second sections. However, church actions do not occur in a vacuum; they may cause the state to react. Thus, the third portion of the chapter examines state responses to church AIDS efforts and places these state responses in the larger context of a dynamic, church-state dialectic in Africa.

The Church-State Relationship and Church Actions on AIDS

Past Church Involvement in Politics

Church participation in politics has waxed and waned since the colonial era when many Catholic and Old Mission Protestant churches helped to implement colonial policies, while the Old African Independent churches were often perceived to challenge the colonial regimes (Gifford 1998). Even though the Catholic and Old Mission churches played a minimal role in the independence struggles—or they came late to the struggle, as the Catholic Church of Angola did—they indirectly affected nationalism through the education of Africa's independence leaders. After independence, some African leaders distanced themselves from these churches because of their past links to colonial regimes (Pobee 1991, 53). Other politicians sought to remake the churches, as Kenneth Kaunda did when he urged Zambian Presbyterians, Methodists, and the Paris Mission to form the United Church of Zambia, whose members then dominated the Kaunda government until the 1980s (Freston 2001). After independence, Catholic and mainline Protestants still had significant influence throughout Africa, particularly in the areas of health and education. They operated the most prestigious schools and many health facilities, and their leaders were linked to the governing elites through shared educational experiences. Yet, in some countries, the Old Independents and New Mission Churches gained favor with post-independence governments (Mugambi 1996). Throughout the 1970s and 1980s as authoritarian regimes came to power throughout the continent, many Catholic, mainline Protestant, and Pentecostal churches remained relatively silent about human rights violations and centralization of power (Ranger 2008).

Samuel Huntington (1991) asserts that churches (particularly the Catholic Church) were crucial in the global spread of democracy in the late 1980s and early 1990s. As a non-state actor that had not been repressed or fully co-opted by African authoritarian leaders, the church (as a collectivity) had the resources, organizational structures, leaders, moral legitimacy, and autonomous arenas of free expression to facilitate democratic movements (Phiri 2000).[1] In a few African countries, such as Malawi where the Catholic bishops issued a pastoral letter that criticized the Hastings Banda regime (Newell 1995), the churches were at the forefront of democratic movements. In the majority of cases, though, churches became involved after students or unions protested against corrupt, authoritarian rulers. As respected, moderate voices, church leaders chaired national conferences to rewrite constitutions, and they acted as mediators between the ruling party and opposition forces (Bratton and van de Walle 1997).

Both Catholics and mainline Protestants channeled their participation in the pro-democracy movements through institutional structures, such as the Catholic bishops or the Protestant ecumenical councils. The Christian Council of Ghana and the country's Catholic bishops criticized President Jerry Rawlings during the 1980s for his government's human rights abuses. Bishop Peter Sarpong, who headed the Catholic Peace and Justice Program, publicly condemned the "wanton killings" of the Rawlings regime and, as early as 1982, called for a constituent assembly to write a new constitution (quoted in Yirenkyi 2000).[2] In 1989, the Catholic Secretariat and the Christian Council issued a joint public statement in which they refused to comply with the regulation that churches register with the Ghanaian government. Such challenges led the Rawlings government to criticize these two religious bodies and to turn to New Independent Churches (primarily neo-Pentecostals) to provide spiritual legitimacy for his regime (Gifford 1998, 2004).

Zambian churches also contributed to the end of Kenneth Kaunda's one-party rule. Before independence, Zambian churches organized into three ecumenical groups, or mother bodies: the Council of Churches in Zambia (composed of mainline Protestants such as the Methodists, Presbyterians, and Anglicans), the Evangelical Fellowship of Zambia (comprised primarily of New Mission Churches that are Pentecostal such as the Assemblies of God), and the Zambia Episcopal Conference (composed of the Catholics). By the 1980s, Kenneth Kaunda had turned from the United Church of Zambia (that he had helped form) to spiritual advisors from Eastern religions. Economic downturn led the Zambian Congress of Trade Unions, and its born-again Christian leader Frederick Chiluba, to demand the end to one-party rule. The mother bodies spoke against the Kaunda government, and they also provided a neutral space where Kaunda and Chiluba could negotiate for multiparty elections. When Chiluba was elected, he appointed members of the Evangelical Fellowship to be his advisors and declared Zambia to be a "Christian nation," a statement that shocked the Council of Churches and the Catholics. While such actions initially gave him favor with various Pentecostal and New Independent churches, Chiluba's increasingly corrupt regime and his attempt to change the constitution to allow him to run for a third term in 2002 led all three mother bodies to mobilize against him (Freston 2001; Ranger 2008).

In probably the most well-known case, the South African Council of Churches issued strong statements against apartheid. While South African black independent churches had a long history of resistance to apartheid, a more collective church movement gained strength in the 1980s, under the leadership of Anglican Bishop Desmond Tutu. By that time, the Catholic Church, inspired by Vatican II and the actions of the Southern African Catholic Bishops' Conference, had joined the anti-apartheid efforts (Brain 1997). With the Kairos Document as an impetus to work for justice, church leaders such as the Reverend Allan Boesak publicly called for the establishment of the United Democratic Front to combine "prophetic Christianity with the liberation struggle"[3] (Walshe 1997, 394). Even though the apartheid regime labeled church leaders as communist stooges and limited attendance at religious services such as funerals, the legitimacy of the churches helped them mobilize local communities and global public opinion against the South African state (Walshe 1997).

Church involvement in politics is not static. With the increased membership in Pentecostal and Old Independent churches such as the Assemblies of God in Zambia, Zionist churches in South Africa and Zimbabwe, and neo-Pentecostal churches in Ghana, mainline Protestants and Catholics have struggled to maintain a prominent political voice. Terence Ranger (2008) argues that African populations increasingly view these mission-established churches to be spiritually dead, elitist, politically opportunistic, and potentially, corrupt.[4] After the move away from one-party rule in several countries in the 1990s, mainline Protestants and Catholics have struggled to redefine their public agenda. In many countries, they have retreated back to social service delivery, including programs to fight AIDS.

In contrast, both the mission-established and new Pentecostal churches have become more involved in politics in the post-Third Wave democratization period. Their political participation has often focused on the narrow issue of moral behavior, particularly in terms of combating corruption and abuse of power by individual leaders. Citizens' perceptions of and experiences with corruption lead them to support the Pentecostal idea of cleansing the public realm of immorality. Religious leaders have urged voters to elect politicians who are morally upstanding and biblically guided Christians, in the hope that these individuals will not become involved in nepotism and corruption (Ranger 2008; Collier 2009). The church background of some recent African political leaders demonstrates the rise of this Christian voice in politics. Ugandan president Yoweri Museveni, former Kenyan president Daniel arap Moi, and former Nigerian president Olusegun Obasanjo all emphasized their born-again Christian backgrounds.[5]

Even with the plethora of African church experiences in politics, it is possible to make three generalizations about the relationship between the involvement of churches in Africa's political development and the response of these churches to AIDS. First, churches with limited political experience have engaged in limited AIDS activities. The lack of political involvement meant that these churches did not learn political strategies or gain issue-based knowledge, and their leaders had few opportunities to gain the organizational skills that could be transferred to AIDS efforts. Second, the Pentecostal emphasis on morality in politics is apparent in these churches' AIDS programs, with their focus on abstinence and marital fidelity. These HIV prevention messages are rooted in an individual orientation to the Gospel, which, as I demonstrate below, is evidenced in their political theology.

Third, there is a correlation between involvement in post-independence democratization movements and early participation in AIDS activities. The Catholic Church was active in democratization efforts in several African countries (as well as globally); it also developed early and comprehensive efforts to fight the disease. Similarly, Protestant ecumenical councils such as the Christian Council of Ghana and the Council of Churches in Kenya were involved in pro-democracy efforts in the 1990s; they also developed early, though more narrow, actions on AIDS (*Nation*, June 4, 1998; *Nation*, November 19, 1998).

It is impossible to say that political involvement in the democratic efforts of the 1990s *caused* churches to act early or comprehensively to combat AIDS. However, church activities on AIDS (or other social issues) do occur in a larger historical context. A few interviewees explained that the process of churches' learning to speak publicly on justice, equality, and human rights in the struggles for democratization made these institutions more aware of the need to address societal problems such as AIDS (Interviews 14, 23, 53). One ecumenical church leader argued that challenging governments on political injustice gave the churches leverage and "made the churches more independent from government" (Interview 25). Churches learned to analyze state actions, to use their moral stature in political debates, and to build coalitions, all skills that church leaders and institutions could transfer to the fight against AIDS. However, while leaders in the Catholic and mainline Protestant churches placed church AIDS activities in the larger historical context of church political mobilization, this was not a theme Pentecostals stressed. Instead, Pentecostals saw their recent political actions (including AIDS activities) as a break with past patterns of mainline and Catholic Church involvement, which they perceived to be corrupt and ineffective.

Political Theology and Actions on AIDS

While a church's activities on AIDS may result from its past political experience, they also may relate to the church's political theology. Political theology can be defined as a religious body's perspectives on state authority, the role of believers in politics, and the relationship between religion and the state (Philpott 2007). Here I analyze three strands in political theology and examine their effects on church AIDS activities. The first emphasizes that church institutions and believers should participate in politics to promote justice, encourage socioeconomic development, and protect human rights (Wolterstorff 2008). While this view acknowledges that corruption, inefficiency, and inequality pervade politics, it also asserts that because Christians are citizens with rights and responsibilities, they cannot ignore politics as a tool for transforming society. Catholic Bishop Peter Sarpong in Ghana explains, "Christ wants his church not to be meaningless in society or to be pushed to the periphery… [but]… to be right at the center of things, right where the action is" (quoted in Yirenkyi 2000, 325). In this view, churches do not take partisan positions, but they work on issues that benefit the common good, such as citizen education, good governance, and peace and reconciliation (Monsma 2001).

As espoused primarily by Catholics and mainline Protestants (particularly Protestant ecumenical councils), these ideas contributed to early church actions to combat AIDS. In the case of the Catholics, those actions often included political advocacy. The African Jesuit AIDS Network illustrated this political theology of engagement when it argued that the church must "advocate for those who have no voice or who may benefit from the moral force of the Church's defence [*sic*] and teaching... and [it must] encourage believers to exercise their responsibility and power as citizens to call on governments for just policies and access to resources" (Czerny and Vitillo 2005-2006, 275). Echoing this statement, a Zambian Catholic claimed that one of the church's roles on AIDS was to "be the prophetic voice," or to emulate the prophets of the Hebrew Bible who challenged political authorities to promote social and economic justice (Interview 23). Similarly, the Christian Councils of Ghana, Kenya, Zimbabwe, South Africa, and Zambia, as well as the All Africa Conference of Churches, have made statements urging political leaders to pay greater attention to AIDS and calling for donors to provide needed AIDS resources (*Catholic Information Service for Africa*, October 12, 2007; *East African Standard*, June 12, 2004; AACC 2008; *Panafrican News Agency*, October 10, 1997). The political theology of engagement informs such actions.

A second strand of political theology asserts that church institutions and Christian believers should divorce themselves from politics. This perspective interprets Jesus Christ's admonition "to render unto Caesar that which is Caesar's" as an instruction to pay taxes and obey laws, but to stay out of politics.[6] Other Christians point to Romans 13, in which the Apostle Paul instructs believers to submit to the political authorities and to concentrate on their spiritual relationship with Christ, as proof that believers should not engage in politics. Zambian Christians who complain that churches are "biblically errant" because they participated in the country's democracy movements exemplify this political theology (Interview 24).

This strand of political theology has prevented churches from engaging in AIDS activities, particularly actions with a public advocacy focus. Some church leaders argue that the only role for the church is to encourage worship, prayer, and Bible study among members, not to educate congregants about social or political issues (such as AIDS) and not to mobilize them for social service provision or advocacy (Interview 37).[7] Some of these churches tended to deny that their members may have AIDS, and they seemed to believe that AIDS only exists among people "outside the church" (Interview 47). If these churches do have AIDS programs, their efforts tend to be narrowly focused, such as small groups of members who provide home-based care for individual congregants. The narrow focus on spirituality over civic engagement and denial of the reality of the presence of AIDS in the community may prevent these churches from acting on the disease.

Churches can change their approach to political theology, a pattern seen among some Pentecostal churches that emulated the theme of political avoidance until the new millennium. Many of these churches adhere to the doctrine of premillennialism, or the general belief that at the end of times, Jesus Christ will return to earth to reign and ultimately, will take believers with him to heaven in the rapture; the doctrine's adherents assert that nonbelievers then will be condemned for eternity. For strict premillennialist Christians, the year 2000 was the year when Jesus would return to earth and the rapture would occur (although not all premillennialists thought the rapture would occur in 2000). As a result, these Christians focused on converting non-believers rather than on worldly issues like socioeconomic development. When the predicted events did not occur, premillennialist Christians began to re-focus their energies on reforming society. Public participation to achieve reforms, though, was often viewed with resignation and a sense of duty. Ugandan pastor Martin Ssempa illustrates: "Politics is a dangerous thing, because power and money are strictly related to corruption. It is not easy for a born-again to move in this setting, but it is necessary." (quoted in Gusman 2009, 74)

This transformation is reflected in a third strand of political theology, which emphasizes Jesus Christ's life and death as the means to save an individual believer from sin. In this political theology, Christ's central act is to forgive an individual's foibles and to empower the believer to live a moral life; Christ's teachings do not primarily demonstrate how to challenge system-level injustices. For those who focus on the believer's personal relationship with Christ, the Christian duty may or may not include participation in politics. The dirtiness of politics—as a realm of compromise, vote trading, and at times, corruption—can taint the believer. However, Christians with this perspective may also hope that believers can bring the good news of rebirth in Christ—and the perceived power of that spiritual rebirth to transform all parts of life—to the realm of politics. The problems of politics are rooted in individual behavior, not institutions or societal structures. According to this view, Christ's redemption can change individual attitudes and actions. Over time, the belief is that these changed hearts and behaviors will enable Christian politicians to reform social structures. Therefore, political participation tends to be narrowly focused on cleaning up politics, not restructuring it (Ranger 2008).[8] This perspective may not threaten the neopatrimonal structures and societal inequalities that exclude some people from political participation and prevent good governance.

This third strand of political theology informs the recent AIDS activities of several established and newer Pentecostal churches. Such participation is narrowly focused on individual-level behavior, such as HIV prevention programs, not structural changes such as greater state funding for health care or better enforcement of laws against domestic violence. While HIV prevention programs are desperately needed to stem the AIDS epidemic, they do not challenge larger social or economic structures such as unemployment, child abuse, or gender-based violence that make HIV prevention problematic. The actions and words of Pastor Ssempa illustrate how the individual salvation emphasis in political theology influences a church to adopt narrowly focused activities on AIDS. Ssempa has organized "abstinence rallies" in Kampala, which are intended to combat what he terms "abstinaphobia," or society's tendency to ostracize youth who abstain from sex before marriage (*Inter Press Service*, June 11, 2004; Ssempa 2009).[9] In contrast, the pastor has made few, if any, statements on how the neopatrimonial politics of the Museveni regime have limited the Ugandan state's ability to grow the economy and provide jobs for unemployed youth (Woodrow Wilson International Center 2005). Since research demonstrates that unemployed youth who are not in school are more likely to engage in sexual relations at an earlier age, a message that calls for both individual sexual responsibility and state responsibilities to youth may not be unreasonable (Whiteside 2005).

These narrowly focused AIDS efforts are situated within a larger social context that stresses that religion, moral behavior, and health are intricately tied together. Focus group participants in Lesotho and Zambia explained that the role of religion is to help individuals, "rather than to seek social change at the public and collective level. Religion connects to morality in terms of personal lifestyle, rather than in terms of political policies" (ARHAP 2006, 78-80). Even when church leaders try to link AIDS to broader themes of social justice, this message may not resonate with ordinary congregants who are hesitant to see churches as a force for political change (Interviews 23, 55).

The tension between these three trends creates ambivalence among Christians about political participation and more narrowly, involvement on AIDS. For example, in a 1995 survey, Ghanaian church members were divided in their responses to the question, "Do you think that clergy should be actively involved in politics (e.g., help to organize political activities, give lectures on government economic programs)?" Forty-one percent said yes, 43 percent said no, and 14 percent were uncertain. Clergy were even less supportive of their own political involvement, with 36 percent answering yes, 43 percent responding no, and 9 percent being uncertain. These numbers may reflect the fact that pastors do not want to divide believers or offend non-Christians with their political involvement (Yirenkyi 2000). Other church leaders fear that if the church involves itself in politics in Africa, it appears to be opportunistically looking for access to state resources (Interview 24). During the 2008 presidential elections, many Ghanaian church leaders seemed cognizant of these problems, when they repeatedly stressed peaceful elections and urged respect for political differences in their public speeches (*Ghanaian Times*, November 12, 2008). In doing so, they avoided partisan leanings.[10]

Ambivalence about political theology shapes church AIDS actions. The same interviewee who argued that the church in Africa must act as a prophetic voice on AIDS also said that the church rarely lived up to this standard (Interview 23). In Ghana, churches which publicly advocated for greater attention to AIDS through the Compassion Campaign were unable to raise adequate funds from congregations to sustain the campaign after donors ended financing (Interviews 30, 35, 50), demonstrating the overall low priority of AIDS advocacy for members. And churches that have publicly stressed sexual morality as a means to combat AIDS often have been silent on the immorality of gender-based violence or discrimination against those with AIDS (Interviews 23, 35, 50; FBO Roundtable 2009).

Finally, one cannot isolate political theology from traditional patterns of African decision making that value consensus building, use praise and proverbs to raise controversial issues, and discourage direct challenges to authority figures (Schaffer 1998). Fear of accusations of witchcraft, which may prevent individuals from being too vocal on issues, also influence the political environment (Berg 2005). During an interview, a Ghanaian church official explained the effect of these traditional norms on church participation in politics and AIDS advocacy:

> If you speak out too strongly on something, you will be named, you will be identified. And forces that you don't even know where they come from will put pressure on you to conform. (Interview 49)
>
> Does this social control [over political debate] exist on the AIDS issue? (Interviewer)
>
> Oh yes! Some are speaking out [on AIDS], but they are not popular, not at all. If you want to succeed in this environment with advocacy, your advocacy has to be information giving: you can use drama, music, radio, educate through publicity; that can be very effective. You can even stage a march where you wear t-shirts and you chant. But you can't agitate or criticize. That is not a part of our culture. (Interview 49)

Differences in cultural norms clearly exist between African societies, with South Africa providing an arena more conductive for activist, vocal organizations that, in the words of the above-cited Ghanaian interviewee, "agitate" (Friedman and Mottair 2004; Johnson 2004). The larger point, though, is that churches are situated within a cultural context. Even churches with a political theology of engagement may tone down their political statements because of cultural expectations for consensus building. For example, annual negotiations between the Zambian government and the Churches Health Association of Zambia (CHAZ) over health priorities and budgets stress consensus building. One CHAZ official explained that CHAZ officers simply go to the president's palace, discuss priorities, and make informal agreements, without acrimony or public argument (FBO Roundtable 2009). For some donors, though, this policy-making process is "too consensual," fostering inefficiency and the belief among all participants that they will materially benefit from their involvement (Interview 13). In sum, churches with a political theology of engagement may be involved on AIDS and use advocacy to shape policies, but they often do so in indirect and informal ways.

Church-State Cooperation in Health Care Provision

Since the colonial period, churches have had a history of cooperation with the state to provide health care, particularly in Anglophone countries. Because of the separation between church and state in France, this secular-religious cooperation on health care provision has been less apparent in former French colonies, where state health care facilities tend to dominate (Cooper 2006).[11] After independence, many mission health care facilities in Africa formed large associations to represent their interests to government and to coordinate programs and finances. For example, the Christian Health Association of Ghana runs 152 health institutions, seventy-eight of which are Catholic and twenty-one, Presbyterian (CHAG 2005). CHAZ runs thirty-two hospitals, fifty-nine rural health centers, and forty-three community clinics (WHO 2005). These associations may cooperate with the state to varying levels, depending on the country. Through a memorandum of understanding, for example, the Zambian government pays the salaries of doctors and nurses who work at CHAZ facilities, while the denominations that are members of CHAZ maintain the health care infrastructure. Both state and CHAZ officials argue that this public-private partnership facilitates provision of health services, particularly in rural areas (Interviews 4, 5, 13, 15).

Churches that acted early, and sometimes comprehensively, to address AIDS were often those with close ties to religious health care providers. Their institutions had access to trusted, first hand information about the effects of AIDS on society. As mentioned in Chapter 2, the experiences that health care workers had with AIDS patients in Salvation Army clinics in Ghana shaped the Christian Council's understanding of AIDS. At regular Christian Council meetings, Salvation Army clinic staff members "passionately" presented compelling stories about people with AIDS (Interview 43). Similar experiences at Catholic clinics and hospitals throughout Africa made it difficult for the Catholic Church hierarchy to ignore the effects of the disease on society. Moreover, churches with links to health care facilities were more likely to engage in policy advocacy on AIDS, even if only behind the scenes. For example, the Zambian mother bodies worked with CHAZ to urge the government to provide free ARV access in 2005 and to remove user fees at private and public health care facilities in 2006 (Interviews 13, 15).[12] In contrast, churches without relations with health care providers, such as some Old and New Independent churches, were less likely to act to fight the disease, particularly during the early years of the epidemic. As some established and neo-Pentecostal churches (particularly urban mega-churches) have become more involved with AIDS in recent years, they have developed relationships with these health care associations. One example is the Expanded Church Response in Zambia, founded by Pentecostal Bishop Joshua Banda of the Northmead Assembly of God, which works closely with CHAZ.

Church-state relations in the area of health care provision demonstrate changing power dynamics. On the one hand, because church health care associations like CHAZ provide needed services that the government either cannot or will not provide, they have some leverage in AIDS policy-making (Interview 2). On the other hand, as a Zambian church leader remarked, "[because] nurses in these church-run institutions are paid by government, unless a church has its own link to outside funding and can pay staff, [it lacks power]" (Interview 10). For many years, the African state and church health care associations worked together with roughly equal power. However, with greater global attention to AIDS and more external funding to faith-based organizations, church health care associations have gained access to more outside resources, as Chapter 5 illustrates. Funding is not only important for programs, but also because it guides policy (Interview 13).

In summary, churches with linkages to health care associations were more likely to act early to address AIDS. The health care associations provided the churches with first hand information on the disease and provided the means through which to develop AIDS programs and to access funding. The fluctuating dynamic between church health care associations and the state creates opportunities for both parties to engage in the fight against AIDS.

Church Representation on AIDS Decision-making Bodies

Because of their political theology, their historic relations with the state, and their role in health care provision, some churches have gained representation on AIDS policy-making institutions in recent years. I do not argue that representation *leads* to church AIDS efforts. Rather, I assert that the development of AIDS policy-making institutions that set priorities and allocate money provides an *opportunity* for churches to sustain their prior AIDS efforts (in the case of the Catholic Church, for example) or to fund new efforts (in the cases of the Northmead Assembly of God or the Makerere Community Church).

Direct church involvement on AIDS policy-making institutions is a relatively new phenomenon, even for churches that established early AIDS programs. According to a survey of AIDS workers, officials at faith-based organizations and policymakers in South Africa, Kenya, and Uganda, many African governments have been slow to include faith-based groups in decision making about approaches to AIDS. Additionally, few religious groups have demanded such representation (Global Health Council 2005). This pattern often resulted because governments considered AIDS to be a technical health issue and situated policy-making and implementation in health ministries. Most African governments did not establish AIDS councils or design multi-sectoral plans until after 2000, when international donors such as the World Bank and UNAIDS provided funding and technical assistance for these efforts (Haven 2005; Putzel 2004).

The Country Coordinating Mechanisms (CCMs) of the Global Fund, developed in 2002, provide a means to assess the level of church representation on one national-level AIDS institution. The Global Fund requires applicant countries to set up a CCM composed of representatives from the government, the donor community, civil society, faith-based organizations, academic institutions, the private sector, and groups that represent people living with HIV/AIDS, TB, and/or malaria. The CCM develops grant proposals and designates principal recipients to oversee grant money and implement the country's program. Principal recipients then provide smaller grants to sub-recipients and help these smaller organizations to monitor and evaluate programs and complete financial records. In 2007, 60 percent of all principal recipients were governments; 17 percent were nongovernmental organizations, community-based associations, faith-based groups, and private sector enterprises; and 12 percent were multilateral donors. (The remaining 11% were unspecified.) (Global Fund 2008c) In terms of funding, 6 percent of grant money globally went to faith-based groups as principal recipients in 2006 (the latest year for available figures), a number that was one-third of all money that civil society principal recipients received (*Boston Globe*, December 1, 2006). In Africa, though, the percentages tended to be higher, with 10.2 percent of funding in southern Africa and 11.8 percent in West and Central Africa going to faith-based organizations (Global Fund 2006b).

I examine the CCMs instead of national AIDS councils because information is more readily available on CCM membership. To be clear, representation does not mean that churches voice concerns, that other decision-makers pay attention to church representatives, or that these religious institutions play more than symbolic roles in these decision-making bodies. For example, some respondents in the aforementioned Global Health Council study reported that church leaders included in AIDS policy-making were sometimes given symbolic roles, such as chairing a country's national AIDS committee, but no real power. A Ugandan participant in the study hinted that the state manipulated church members in these institutions: "Sometimes [churches] have been used as a rubber stamp" (Global Health Council 2005, 66). Despite these problems, representation does at least provide an opportunity for churches to shape AIDS policy and resource allocation.

Table 4.1 provides the percentage and number of seats on the CCM that Christian and non-Christian faith-based organizations held in

Christian-majority countries in 2009. I use indigenous Christian faith-based organizations, not international faith-based groups such as World Vision, as an indicator for churches, because individual denominations rarely have representation on a CCM. The table demonstrates that countries vary in the level of representation of Christian faith-based organizations from 13 percent in the Democratic Republic of Congo to 0 percent in Ethiopia and Congo-Brazzaville. The mean rate of representation for Christian faith-based organizations is 5 percent, higher than the global average of 4 percent for all CCMs (*Boston Globe*, December 1, 2006). Since the CCMs must include a variety of representatives from numerous sectors, the average does not seem extremely low.

Table 4.1 provides the names of principal recipients that are faith-based organizations and lists the funding round in which those organizations received money. Despite the fact that most of the twenty-three Christian-majority countries listed have some form of church health care associations (although not all associations combine Protestant and Catholic facilities), only three of these countries had faith-based organizations as principal recipients by 2009, and only CHAZ and the Zimbabwe Association of Church Hospitals were explicitly Christian. CHAZ is unique because it has received grants in three separate rounds of funding.

Representation on the relatively new CCMs has enabled churches to sustain programming and to lobby for new initiatives. For example, as the representative for all faith-based organizations on the Zambian CCM and as a principal recipient, CHAZ has been able to access funds to sustain and expand its AIDS programs and to support new church initiatives, such as the Expanded Church Response. Similarly, Ssempa's Campus Alliance to Wipe Out AIDS received 34 million shillings (approximately $18,500 in 2006) as a sub-recipient of Global Fund money. In an event that seemed to hint at Ssempa's connections to the CCM, Global Fund Board members made a specific visit to the Campus Alliance in 2006 and praised its financial accountability and creative programs (*New Vision*, January 13, 2006). Church involvement in policy-making and funding decisions is not without potential challenges. One is that not all church organizations may want to be a principal recipient. While control over resources (which then drives policy) may be inviting, principal recipients often need to accept a broader approach to AIDS (particularly in terms of HIV prevention) than some churches may be willing to accept.

Table 4.1 Representation of Faith-Based Organizations on CCMs in Christian-Majority Countries

Country	Total CCM Members	% Christian FBOs	# Christian FBOs	% Other FBOs	# Other FBOs	FBO Principal Recipients
Angola	26	4	1	0	0	none
Botswana	22	5	1	0	0	none
Burundi	28	7	2	4	1	none
Cameroon	50	4	2	2	1	none
Central African Republic	45	7	3	2	1	none
Congo-Brazzaville	23	0	0	4	1	none
Democratic Republic of Congo	40	13	5	3	1	none
Eritrea	15	7	1	0	0	none
Ethiopia	14	0	0	7	1	Ethiopian Inter-Faith Forum for Development (Round 7)
Gabon	32	3	1	6	2	none
Ghana	29	3	1	0	0	none
Kenya	25	8	2	4	1	none
Lesotho	25	4	1	4	1	none
Malawi	19	5	1	0	0	none
Namibia	28	4	1	4	1	none
Rwanda	27	4	1	4	1	none
Sao Tome & Principe	33	3	1	0	0	none
South Africa	14	7	1	0	0	none
Swaziland	31	6	2	0	0	none
Tanzania	21	10	2	5	1	none
Uganda	58	2	1	2	1	none
Zambia	22	5	1	5	1	CHAZ (Rounds 1, 4, 8)
Zimbabwe	20	5	1	5	1	Zimbabwe Association of Church Related Hospitals (Round 5)

NOTE: I omitted Cape Verde, Equatorial Guinea, and Seychelles because they had no CCMs at the time of research.

Source: Global Fund 2010a.

For example, in debates on the Uganda CCM about who would serve as the civil society principal recipient in the country's 2010 application, church leaders were willing to cede this role to The AIDS Support Organization (TASO): "We knew if we were a principal recipient, we would have to get into issues about condoms and other things that some of our members would not want us to support." (Uganda Religious Leaders 2010)

An additional challenge is that church involvement in policy-making and funding decisions introduces a new power dynamic into the relationship that church health care associations have with their constituent denominations and individual congregations. Sometimes constituent members have assumed that because of common theological beliefs or church loyalties, member churches will receive money through their representatives on the CCM. In Zambia, some respondents explained that CHAZ constituent members often do not understand the complex reality of the CCM's funding decisions. The CCM is concerned about giving funds to churches that can achieve specific objectives. While some churches have the capacity to oversee AIDS programs, wisely use funds, and monitor and evaluate programs, others lack such capacity but still think that they deserve grants. One individual explained that as soon as CHAZ became a principal recipient, "Every church in Zambia—from the biggest to the smallest—wanted money." When some of these churches did not get grants, "They did not understand that they needed to have program plans and systems to oversee grant monies" (CHAZ 2009). Denial of grants to constituent members can have a cost. Other church-based AIDS program coordinators hinted that CHAZ's rejection of funding applications has angered some of its member churches (Interviews 1, 10).

This first section has examined how four components of the church-state relationship may influence church actions on AIDS. First, churches with prior actions in politics were among those to first act on AIDS. In contrast, Pentecostal churches have more recently addressed the disease and have tended to frame AIDS policies in the ways they approach politics, through the lens of individual moral behavior. Second, churches with a political theology of engagement and, third, links to health care institutions have often acted early and (sometimes) comprehensively on AIDS. Finally, church representation on CCMs enables churches to access funds for their efforts, although not all churches are on the CCMs and if they are, not all benefit materially from this position.

Political and Social Context: An Opportunity for Church Actions?

The social movement literature demonstrates that "changes or differences in the political and institutional environment" can influence mobilization (van Stekelenburg and Kandermans 2009, 25). Such opportunities as changes in state power, economic transitions, and the rise of new global issues may create moments in which movements can organize (Tarrow 1989). While resources (such as leadership) and state policies may shape this mobilization, the larger context also facilitates and limits these actions (Ondetti 2006). While the next chapter examines the opportunity structures of increased global attention to AIDS, this section concentrates on the ways a country's level of political openness and its level of inter-church competition correlate with its churches' actions on AIDS.

To assess the influence of these two contextual factors, I look at aggregate responses to the disease by all churches in the twenty-three Christian-majority countries with HIV prevalence data (see Table 1.1). The level of analysis is the country and the unit of analysis is all churches in that country. I approach the problem thusly because I want to discern how the national political and religious environment may shape church AIDS actions. To determine a country's aggregate level of church responses to AIDS, I use four indicators: (1) a country's number of newspaper stories on AIDS and churches between 1995 and 2008; (2) the number of national church organizations that participate in global ecumenical AIDS efforts; (3) the number of times that UNAIDS mentioned churches and/or faith-based organizations in its 2008 reports of specific countries; and (4) the number of church leaders as of 2006 who participated in ANERELA+.

Newspaper articles provide a general sense of church activity on AIDS, although I acknowledge that this is a crude measure (see Chapter 2 for the limits of using newspapers as a data source). The level of church participation in the ecumenical AIDS efforts of the Ecumenical Advocacy Alliance, the World Council of Churches, the All Africa Conference of Churches, and the World Evangelical Alliance gives some indication of how willing churches are to cooperate internationally, to advocate on the global level, and to learn from other churches. (Chapter 5 provides more information on these organizations.) Inclusion of churches in UNAIDS reports provides an external evaluation of church involvement. ANERELA+ membership broadly indicates how seriously a country's church leaders view AIDS and how much they will mobilize to support people with the disease.[13] I do not include the percentage of CCM seats that Christian faith-based organizations hold because this number indicates how willing government is to bring churches into policy-making, not how proactive churches themselves are on AIDS. However, in the case of countries where churches are principal recipients, I take that fact into account. I acknowledge that these are rough indicators and that it can be difficult to compare some data (such as UNAIDS reports) across countries. My goal is to discern broad patterns in Christian-majority countries, not to provide exact measures of church efforts.

I categorize countries as having high, medium, or low levels of church response to AIDS. High-level response countries had over eight hundred news articles on churches and AIDS between 1995 and 2008, over fifty pastors in ANERELA+, at least two references to church AIDS efforts in a country's UNAIDS report, and participation in ecumenical AIDS efforts. If a country had an overabundance of news articles and a large number of ANERELA+ members, but no UNAIDS mentions, I gave extra weight to news articles and ANERELA+ participation, since these were the most objective indicators of the four. Using these criteria, Kenya, South Africa, Uganda, Zambia, and Zimbabwe had high response levels. These countries vary in the severity of their epidemics.

Medium-level response countries had five hundred to eight hundred news articles and between twenty and fifty national church leaders in ANERELA+. They had sporadic participation in ecumenical AIDS efforts. If the UNAIDS 2008 report mentions churches, it does so in a general way and situates church efforts within broader civil society AIDS responses. Again, I allow some flexibility in my country classifications. For example, Tanzania had seventy ANERELA+ members, but no specific church mentions in the UNAIDS report and little published participation in global ecumenical AIDS efforts. Ghana had over five hundred news articles, but only fifteen ANERELA+ members. Yet, its churches are quite involved in global ecumenical AIDS efforts. The countries in this category are Botswana, Ethiopia, Ghana, Lesotho, Malawi, Namibia, Rwanda, and Tanzania. Again, they vary in their HIV prevalence.

Low-level countries had fewer than three hundred news articles, fewer than twenty ANERELA+ members, limited or no participation in ecumenical efforts, and no mention of churches in the UNAIDS report. These countries are Angola, Burundi, Cameroon, Central African Republic, Congo-Brazzaville, Democratic Republic of Congo, Eritrea, Equatorial Guinea, Gabon, and Swaziland. Table 4.2 classifies Christian-majority countries by high, medium, and low levels of church responses to AIDS. The table also includes each country's epidemic type, its Freedom House classification for political and civil rights, and the percentage of the population that is Catholic. I use the latter two indicators below.[14]

I now question how a country's political and religious context might shape church AIDS responses. First, I hypothesize that churches in countries with greater political freedoms will be more likely than churches in less free countries to have AIDS programs and to advocate on AIDS. In theory, elections in systems that protect political and civil rights should hold leaders accountable for AIDS spending. Freedom of the press should enable citizens and churches to access information on AIDS programs. Freedom of association should enable civil society groups such as churches to influence state AIDS policies (Siegle, Weinstein, and Halperin 2004).

I use information from Table 4.2 to tabulate the number of countries with low, medium, and high levels of church AIDS response in the not free, partly free, and free political contexts. The results are provided in Table 4.3, which controls for epidemic type. A few generalizations can be made from the table, although overall, it is inconclusive. First, churches in all five free countries have engaged in high or medium levels of response, regardless of the epidemic type. No free country has churches with a low level of response. Second, seven of the nine countries in the not free category have low levels of church response. Only one country in the not free category—Zimbabwe, a country with a history of church activism—has a high level of church response to AIDS (Mukonyora 2008). Third, nine of the fifteen countries with low-level epidemics have low levels of church response, an outcome which does not relate directly to the political environment but may show that churches respond to pressing issues, and in low HIV prevalence environments, AIDS may not have much saliency. However, the corollary—that churches in high prevalence countries should have high levels of response—was not evident. Only three of eight countries with high-level epidemics have high-level church responses, a fact that may reflect the reality that church responsiveness to AIDS varies based on several factors I have analyzed, including organizational resources, biblical frameworks, and church-state history.

Table 4.2 Level of Aggregate Church AIDS Response in Christian-Majority Countries, with Epidemic Type, Freedom House Classification, and Catholic Population

Country	Epidemic Type	Freedom House Classification	Catholic Population (% total)
High-Level Church Response			
Kenya	generalized, low level	partly free	24
South Africa	generalized, high level	free	8
Uganda	generalized, low level	partly free	42
Zambia	generalized, high level	partly free	33
Zimbabwe	generalized, high level	not free	9
Medium-Level Church Response			
Botswana	generalized, high level	free	3
Ethiopia	generalized, low level	partly free	1
Ghana	generalized, low level	free	9
Lesotho	generalized, high level	free	45
Malawi	generalized, high level	partly free	25
Namibia	generalized, high level	free	18
Rwanda	generalized, low level	not free	57
Tanzania	generalized, low level	partly free	24
Low-Level Church Response			
Angola	generalized, low level	not free	55
Burundi	generalized, low level	partly free	62
Cameroon	generalized, low level	not free	26
Central African Republic	generalized, high level	partly free	29
Congo-Brazzaville	generalized, low level	not free	62
Democratic Republic of Congo	generalized, low level	not free	55
Eritrea	generalized, low level	not free	13
Equatorial Guinea	generalized, low level	not free	86
Gabon	generalized, low level	partly free	61
Swaziland	generalized, high level	not free	25

Note: Cape Verde, Sao Tome and Principe, and Seychelles are omitted because of a lack of HIV data.

Source: Freedom House 2009; UNAIDS 2008b; US Department of State 2008a; author calculations of Catholic percentages from Table 1.4.

The generally inconclusive evidence of Table 4.3 is in keeping with prior research that has not demonstrated a strong relationship between Freedom House scores and civil society representation on CCMs or between Freedom House scores and health spending (Patterson 2006). Perhaps these inconclusive results demonstrate that in democracies the "tyranny of the majority," particularly if that majority stigmatizes people with AIDS and/or denies the disease, may prevent churches from AIDS actions. The negative reactions of American churches to AIDS when the disease first emerged in the United States in the early 1980s demonstrated that a democratic context does not necessarily make it easier for religious bodies (or civil society in general) to respond positively to AIDS. In fact, free media coverage and open public debate on AIDS probably increased hysteria in the United States and prevented some churches from addressing the problem (Siplon 2002; Beckley and Koch 2002).

Table 4.3 Level of Aggregate Church Response and Country Freedom, Controlling for Epidemic Type in Christian-Majority Countries

	Freedom House Classification		
Epidemic Type	Not Free	Partly Free	Free
Generalized, High-Level Epidemic (N=8)			
High-Level Response (3)	1	1	1
Medium-Level Response (4)	0	1	3
Low-Level Response (1)	1	0	0
Generalized, Low-Level Epidemic (N=15)			
High-Level Response (2)	0	2	0
Medium-Level Response (4)	1	2	1
Low-Level Response (9)	6	3	0
	N= 9	N= 9	N= 5

Source: Compiled by author from information in Table 4.2.

Even though there is limited evidence of an overall correlation between political freedom and levels of church responses to AIDS, this finding does not mean that such freedoms are inconsequential at the individual country level. In Ghana, for example, the Catholics and mainline Protestants became publicly active on AIDS only after the 2000 election, which the chosen successor of Jerry Rawlings, the former military dictator, lost. Alternation in power provided an opportunity for churches to advocate on AIDS and gain the attention of a new government (Patterson 2006). On the other hand, even though the Zimbabwean government has repressed church leaders (particularly Anglicans), many churches have been active on AIDS (US Department of State 2008b). UNAIDS partially credited the HIV prevention programs of religiously based organizations with helping to bring down Zimbabwe's HIV prevalence (*Herald*, December 8, 2005; UNAIDS 2005b). And as illustrated above, the Global Fund granted money to the Zimbabwe Association of Church Related Hospitals for its AIDS response. The lack of democracy in Zimbabwe has not prevented church AIDS efforts.

Table 4.2 reinforces the aforementioned point that countries with high levels of church response tend to be countries where the church has been or currently is active in promoting democracy, human rights, and government accountability (Ranger 2008; Gifford 1998; Freston 2001). Churches in South Africa, Kenya, Zimbabwe, and Zambia were active in the struggle against authoritarianism, although churches in Uganda have only recently challenged President Museveni's power centralization, particularly with his removal of presidential term limits (Uganda Religious Leaders 2010; Mwenda 2004; Freston 2001).[15] Similarly, Ghana, a free country with a history of church involvement in politics, has a low-level epidemic but it is classified with a medium level of church responses to AIDS. Other countries with medium-level church responses in low-level epidemic countries (Rwanda, Ethiopia, and Tanzania) do not have the same history of church political involvement. In fact, the church in Rwanda was indicted for its implicit and explicit participation in the 1994 genocide. Thus, the relationship between past political activity and AIDS efforts does not hold in all cases.

In addition to the growing political pluralism in Africa after the Cold War, diversity in Christian congregations in the last generation has also increased. How has this change affected churches' actions on AIDS? Will the fear of losing members to other churches in a religiously competitive environment influence how (or if) churches address controversial issues such as AIDS? Assuming that churches seek to maximize their membership and the financial resources needed to run their organizations, Anthony Gill (1998) examines the effect of increasing religious competition in Latin America in the 1960s and 1970s on Catholic Church opposition to authoritarian rule. By the 1960s, Protestant churches in countries such as El Salvador and Brazil had attracted thousands of former Catholics as members, particularly among the poor who suffered the most under authoritarian regimes (Martin

1990). Gill argues that because of the increased religious competition, the Catholic Church responded to the perception that it was an apologist for authoritarian rule and began to distance itself from the state and call for democracy.

I define a religiously competitive country as one where no Christian denomination has a majority. Since the Catholic Church is the largest single denomination (Protestants comprise many denominations), I define countries with a Catholic majority as not religiously competitive and those without a Catholic majority to be competitive. Because of Protestant diversity, countries without a Catholic majority most likely do not have a single Protestant denomination with a majority. I hypothesize that in countries without a Catholic majority (i.e., countries that are more religiously competitive), churches will be more likely to address AIDS. To be relevant, churches in religiously competitive environments need to address issues pertinent in the lives of their members. Given the high HIV prevalence levels in many Christian countries, and the assertion that African Christians are partially attracted to churches which address their congregants' material needs (Jenkins 2007), I assume AIDS activities enable churches to reach out to new members and to meet the needs of their current parishioners. Conversely, I hypothesize that countries with a Catholic majority (i.e., those that are less religiously competitive) will have churches that are less likely to act on AIDS.

Table 4.4 shows that among the sixteen countries without a Catholic majority (i.e., countries that are religiously competitive), five had a high level of church response to AIDS, seven had a medium level, and four had a low level. Among the seven countries with a Catholic majority (i.e., those with less religious competition), six had a low level of church response to AIDS and one had a medium level of response. There are no Catholic-majority countries with a high level of church response to AIDS.

On first glance, these trends seem to indicate that in religiously competitive environments churches are more likely to address AIDS. They also seem to problematize the assertion of Chapter 2 that the Catholic Church developed the earliest and most comprehensive AIDS programs. To unpack this conundrum, it is important to acknowledge that there are two factors occurring in the data: religious competition and epidemic type. As demonstrated in terms of the political environment, countries with low-level epidemics have churches with lower levels of AIDS responses. It just happens that six of the ten countries with low-level church responses have a Catholic majority. It is impossible to discern whether it is the lack of religious competition, the low-level epidemic, or other factors that lead to less church activity on AIDS. This finding does not distract from the fact that the Catholic Church is one of many church actors involved in AIDS in southern Africa, a region with Christian diversity.

Table 4.4 Level of Aggregate Church Response and Catholic Majority, Controlling for Epidemic Type in Christian-Majority Countries

	Catholic Majority	
Epidemic Type	Yes	No
Generalized, High-Level Epidemic (N=8)		
High-Level Response (3)	0	3
Medium-Level Response (4)	0	4
Low-Level Response (1)	0	1
Generalized, Low-Level Epidemic (N=15)		
High-Level Response (2)	0	2
Medium-Level Response (4)	1	3
Low-Level Response (9)	6	3
	N= 7	N= 16

Source: Compiled by author from information in Table 4.2.

To better appreciate why the level of religious competition in a country has no clear influence on church AIDS efforts, it is important to recognize that church membership is based on multiple factors, including family ties, socialization, peer pressure, class identity, emotional attachment, worship style preferences, location, and church doctrine (Hoge and Carroll 1978). In the African context where maintaining communal ties and keeping the peace are crucial, social pressures to remain in a religious community may be strong. Even if members do not agree with church actions on AIDS (or other issues), they may not act as market agents and leave a church to join another. The religious competition argument also does not fully hold up because church actions which may not seem popular, such as AIDS activities, may be rooted in biblical principles, not rational calculations about attracting members (Philpott 2007).

An ecumenical church leader argued that if a church is really committed to its biblical mission, and it sees its role as providing leadership to address important social problems, it should not care about what other churches are doing on any issue:

> I would hope that we would never think that we should not speak on issues like injustice, bad governance, health, or disease and only focus on the spiritual, personal aspects of faith [because other churches are only doing that]. For us, faith isn't just those personal, Sunday morning aspects. To be saved means being the salt and light of the community. It is who we are. (Interview 53)

Thus, the religious competition explanation, just like the openness of a country's political environment, does not sufficiently explicate church AIDS actions. This is because, as I outline in this book's other chapters, other factors matter and because church activity does not occur in a vacuum. As the next section shows, state responses may further influence church actions on AIDS.

The Church-State Dialectic: State Responses to Church AIDS Activities

Having examined how the church-state relationship may influence church AIDS activities, I now outline five overall patterns in state reactions to these church activities. I then use the Zambia case to highlight these. The first response is ignoring or downplaying the church's voice in AIDS policy-making, an action made possible by the relative weakness of civil society. Although churches may be more powerful than many civil society institutions in Africa, they still may lack resources, strong leadership, political sophistication, and organization—all factors that increase civil society power in its interactions with the state (Michael 2004). Even though belief in the power of spiritual forces pervades Africa, religious *institutions* or their leaders may not always be perceived to have power. It may be easy for the state to ignore or downplay the church's voice in AIDS policy-making, just as it can ignore other civil society groups involved with the issue. One Zambian interviewee situated churches within a context of civil society and then explained, "If civil society sends its information to government or tries to advocate using its information, government rarely pays much attention to it unless civil society has a multilateral agency to support it, like UNAIDS.... [Civil society advocacy and research] are rarely appreciated" (Interview 18). The respondent illustrated not only that government ignores civil society, but also that civil society's weakness requires it to rely on international organizations to get government's attention.

Second, the state may exclude civil society groups from decision-making venues. Churches have complained that they have not been brought into decisions about HIV prevention programs, particularly condom distribution and advertisement campaigns (Pfeiffer 2004; Interview 9). Sometimes the state has had to retreat from such policies, paying the price for not engaging churches in decision making. One ecumenical leader explained: "When the state does not consult the church leadership, it encounters resistance" (Interview 25). However, this is not always the case. Ghanaian churches, despite representation on the Ghana AIDS Commission Steering Committee, have had little influence on the Commission's decision to incorporate a comprehensive HIV prevention message that includes the message of condom use. While some church leaders are pragmatic about condoms (Interviews 35, 41, 49), others are strongly against them (Interview 33). Because the government has a pro-condom position, "The head of GAC [the Ghana AIDS Commission] is not very popular with churches" (Interview 47).

Third, the state may try to co-opt the church or to limit its actions on AIDS. The state may adopt this strategy because church involvement can "make the government very uncomfortable" (Interview 25). We have seen that churches respond to AIDS with material programs (e.g., care, support, and treatment efforts) and through spiritual interventions (e.g., prayer, healing, and fellowship). The state may seek to control actions in both arenas. In response to churches' material activities, state officials may limit church access to AIDS funds or prevent their representation on decision-making boards. One respondent hinted that some Nigerian churches' participation had been compromised since church leaders receive "tokens of appreciation" such as cars and office space from the state. As a result, those church leaders have been hesitant to challenge state decisions (Interview 2).

The state also may attempt to control how the church uses its spiritual responses to AIDS. Because the line between the sacred and secular is murky, the state may make incursions into the religious realm. While pluralists often view the state as autonomous and devoid of cultural influences, state incorporation of spirituality shows the inadequacy of this assumption (Thomas 2005). The state's objective may reflect politicians' fear that religious leaders will access the powerful, spiritual realm to negatively affect these political officials (Ellis and ter Haar 2004; Meyer 2004). State reactions may be a response to the increased attraction of spiritual healing ceremonies, prayer camps, witchcraft accusations, and false prophets which have accompanied Africa's increase in AIDS cases and the continent's limited access to ARVs. A few examples illustrate this trend. In March 2008, the Malawian legislature debated a law which would make it illegal for individuals, including traditional healers and churches, to claim they can cure AIDS. In Kenya, the government requires registration of traditional healers in order to curtail people from asserting their ability to cure AIDS. An editorial in the *Mmegi/Reporter* (March 27, 2008) urged the government in Botswana to copy Kenya and Malawi's actions.

These actions may appear to be negative attacks on religious freedom, but on the positive side, some state attempts to control church AIDS responses may help to protect citizens. For example, the Democratic Republic of Congo's 2006 constitution explicitly prohibits accusing children of sorcery (*Human Rights Watch News,* April 1, 2006), a reaction to an increased number of children blamed for witchcraft.[16] Child welfare agencies estimate that as many as 70 percent of Kinshasa's street children have been accused of witchcraft (*Human Rights Watch News,* April 1, 2006). Many are AIDS orphans who have lost family property and have been pushed from their homes (*Angola Press Agency*, September 2, 2007; *UN Integrated Regional Information Networks*, December 12, 2006). Some churches have sought to cure these "child witches" by withholding food, imprisoning them, and/or beating them. Such actions are rooted in the belief that "child sorcerers have the power to transmit any disease, including AIDS" (*UN Integration Regional Information Networks*, April 21, 2005). Clearly, state attempts to control such religious activities promote child welfare.

Fourth, the state may capitulate to church pressure for policy changes on AIDS. Such outcomes have been more likely to occur when the church could link the disease to the message of sexual morality, since (as demonstrated above) the general population tends to view such linkages to be legitimate. This pattern is evident in churches' ability to pressure the state and donors to limit condom campaigns, particularly condom advertisements. Churches in Angola, Zambia, Malawi, Mozambique, Kenya, Ghana, and Swaziland have criticized government condom campaigns for encouraging sexual promiscuity and for being sexually explicit (*UN Integrated Regional Information Network*, July 27, 2001). In a particularly vivid quote, a Swazi pastor said, "Even if you are a religious person, pastor or a priest, you cannot help but get sexually aroused by the explicit visual materials they distribute" (*African Eye News Service,* April 17, 2001). Because of church actions, governments and donor agencies have removed television and billboard condom advertisements or toned down their sexual content (*African*

Church Information Service, June 24, 2002; *East African Standard*, November 28, 2006; Interviews 7, 9).

Churches also have influenced national HIV prevention programs, particularly in terms of school curriculum. The importance of church-funded schools in Anglophone Africa gives the churches influence on education issues. Kenya's Catholics lobbied for the AIDS curriculum at secondary schools to include abstinence messages (*Nation*, July 22, 2000). When Ugandan churches reacted negatively to sex education programs in primary and secondary schools (*Monitor*, February 6, 2002), the government developed its curriculum on abstinence and fidelity which downplayed condom use (Human Rights Watch 2005).

Fifth, state officials have sought to situate AIDS actions in light of religious metaphors and messages of biblical morality. In 2000, then Ugandan Vice President Specioza Kazibwe urged the Catholic Church to accept condoms in the AIDS fight. She argued that her Catholic faith made her believe that God wanted the church to help people live a healthy life (*Monitor*, June 22, 2000). She used the Christian message that God wants his people to flourish and the Catholic emphasis on holistic development (the idea that both physical and spiritual health matter) to challenge the Catholic Church's policy against condoms. Moreover, by discussing her own Catholic background, the vice president sought to legitimate her moral claims.

The Zambia Case

Church-state interactions on AIDS must be situated in the context of Zambia's larger constitutional reform process. In 2007, the three Christian mother bodies tried to influence the process for re-writing the country's constitution (*Times of Zambia*, October 12, 2007; October 25, 2007; November 20, 2007; November 29, 2007; January 8, 2008). They formed the Oasis Forum, a broad organization of civic groups and churches, which was headed by the leader of the Christian Council of Zambia, African Methodist Episcopal pastor Suzanne Matale. The Oasis Forum demanded that then President Levy Mwanawasa set up a representative constituent assembly to re-write the country's constitution and that civil society groups choose their own representatives for the assembly. In several public battles with the president, the Oasis Forum challenged Mwanawasa's plan to have the legislature choose the constituent assembly members. Some of this advocacy included public protests during the Southern African Development Community meeting held in Lusaka (*Post*, August 16, 2007; *Times of Zambia*, August 13, 2007).

When the Oasis Forum was unable to influence the constitutional review process, it decided to boycott the constituent assembly. However, some churches in the mother bodies, including the large Assemblies of God, criticized this decision, and a number even withdrew from these national councils (*Times of Zambia*, January 8, 2008). Several popular Pentecostal leaders, including Bishop Banda, decided to participate in the constitutional review process. In contrast, the Catholics and the Christian Council still had not joined the convention as of late 2009. In March 2009, the Catholic bishops issued a pastoral letter, in which they criticized the government for economic problems, corruption, and "a constitution-making process that is still controversial and seems not to be in the interest of citizens" (*Ecumenical News International*, March 11, 2009). Similarly, the Oasis Forum and the Patriotic Front (the party which lost the October 2008 presidential election by 2 percent) continued to criticize the constitutional process.

What does this larger context mean for the ways that the Zambian state has dealt with churches on AIDS? First, the pattern of sidelining or ignoring churches is evident in the fact that the Christian Council and the Catholic bishops have not been major voices in AIDS institutions, such as the National HIV/AIDS/STI/TB Council (NAC). While it is impossible to say that these churches' marginalization is a result of their challenges to the constitutional review process, several interviewees emphasized that any civil society action on AIDS could not be understood without situating it within the larger battle between the state and the Oasis Forum (Interviews 5, 10, 13, 20, 21).

Second, some religious and secular AIDS officials would argue that state co-optation and control of churches is apparent. One church official said, "Now some churches have been corrupted by government so they don't speak out on government [AIDS] policy. But sometimes if other churches speak out against the government then the government will [shut] them out" (Interview 14). Some individuals assert that Banda is one of those church leaders that government has co-opted. His critics perceive that his appointment to the NAC is a reward for his support for the constitutional convention (Interview 10). Nicolas van de Walle (2001) argues that in many cases, presidential commissions and committees are the means through which state officials disperse patronage to supporters and build networks to keep themselves in power. As an arena to set policy and guide resource distribution, AIDS councils throughout Africa exemplify this type of institution.

These appointments may provide churches some access to power and resources, but not enough to really influence policies. In the case of Zambia's NAC, several informants said it was a relatively weak institution in terms of policy-making and implementation (Interviews 12, 20, 21). One critic commented: "To say that NAC is coordinating is a bit inaccurate" (Interview 18). Established by the parliament in 2002, the NAC is not an independent body situated within the Office of the President or Vice President. Instead, it must report to the Ministry of Health, which has the ultimate say on AIDS policies. The Council cannot hold the other line ministries accountable for their AIDS policies, and the Council's role is often unclear (NAC 2005, 4; Interviews 4, 5, 6, 13). Additionally, its budget is quite small in comparison to the large amount of AIDS funds coming into the country. In 2007, donors and the government spent approximately $400 million on AIDS, with donors providing roughly 90 percent of this amount. The NAC, which is supposed to coordinate all of the AIDS funding, had a budget of roughly $6 million (Interview 13). For those who agree with van de Walle's perspective, inclusion of churches into the NAC could be a relatively cheap and easy way for the government to co-opt religious voices.

Examining Banda's position on the NAC from another angle, however, one can see a third pattern—one in which the state appreciates (if not capitulates to) the church. The bishop and his congregation have considerable experience developing AIDS programs. Also, this religious leader's popularity and charisma, his links to external donors, his leadership of the Expanded Church Response, and his participation in the global network of Assemblies of God churches give him and his congregation a certain level of legitimacy and autonomy on the AIDS issue. The state needs these societal leaders and experts on the NAC for the institution to gain legitimacy in the eyes of citizens and donors.

Zambian churches appear to play both roles. The Northmead Assembly of God may be somewhat co-opted, but it also has shaped government HIV prevention programs and particularly, condom messages. Even the apparent marginalization of the Catholic bishops and the Christian Council from the NAC does not fully limit their influence in AIDS decision making. Instead, these churches are represented in policy-making and resource allocation on the CCM through CHAZ, since the Catholic and mainline Protestant churches run most of the CHAZ-related hospitals and clinics. The murkiness of these power relations in Zambia demonstrates the complexity of state-church interactions on many issues, not just AIDS. Vertical, personalized ties link the high politics of state institutions with the low politics of church congregations and the spiritual realm. Patrick Chabal and Jean Pascal Daloz (1999, 28) write, "Most political actors are simultaneously dominant and dominated, one of the links in one of the many chains of dependence." The civil society literature often understates these webs of both dependence and power, since it segregates civil society associations from the state. The complicated relationship between the Zambian state and the country's churches challenges this perspective.

Conclusion

A central theme of this chapter has been the complex and dynamic relationship between churches and the state. This relationship is manifested in historical interactions, political theology, state-church cooperation in health care provision, and church representation on the CCMs. The state-church nexus influences how and when churches addressed AIDS, with churches that acted early building on their past political experiences, a political theology of engagement, and their work in health care provision. Churches that have become involved in AIDS more recently have tended to be relatively new to the political arena, and they have often viewed the disease and politics in terms of individual morality.

There is limited evidence that a democratic political context encourages churches to act on AIDS. Similarly, churches do not seem to be influenced by the fear that they will gain or lose members in a religiously competitive environment if they develop AIDS programs. A country's type of epidemic may play as big a role as its political and religious context in determining church AIDS activities. Some churches that have responded to the disease have gained representation on CCMs to solidify their access to resources. In their interactions with the state, external resources can become a source of power for churches, as can churches' ability to use moral arguments and their links to the spiritual realm. As the next chapter illustrates, these abilities are situated in a larger context, one in which global factors often shape church efforts to fight the pandemic.

---

[1] In some African countries, churches were co-opted by authoritarian leaders. Two examples are Rwanda and Liberia (Gifford 1998; Longman 2010). My broader point is that in comparison to most other African civil society organizations, the church had more independence and resources (Joseph 1993).

[2] A new Ghanaian constitution was not written until 1992.

[3] Written in Soweto in 1985 by an ecumenical group of pastors, the Kairos Document challenged the church to address apartheid. It criticized the mainline churches for being unwilling to directly combat apartheid, and it situated the role of churches in the apartheid struggle in a larger political and social context. While very controversial, the document galvanized churches.

[4] In the *Ghanaian Times* (October 20, 2008), a Presbyterian pastor echoed this theme when he complained that his denomination is "not spiritually inclined," a fact which he argued hampers church growth.

[5] One could question the morality of these leaders' regimes in terms of corruption and human rights abuses. My point is not to assess this morality, but to illustrate that these leaders have claimed legitimacy and moral purity because of their Christian faith.

[6] See Matthew 22:15-21.

[7] Some pastors at the Network for African Congregational Theology Conference on Churches, Poverty, and AIDS made this argument. Author observation, Lusaka, Zambia, August 4-11, 2007.

[8] As the rise of evangelical candidates, voters, and interest groups in the United States demonstrates, many American evangelicals have embraced this third perspective on political theology. For many (although not all), moral issues such as abortion or gay marriage motivate political participation (Guth et al. 2006).

[9] On his website, Ssempa remarks, "If there is such a thing as homophobia, then there is such a thing as abstinaphobia." As Chapter 5 argues, Ssempa's remarks exemplify an increasing challenge to the global AIDS regime from some African churches (Ssempa 2009).

[10] Some of my Ghanaian colleagues, however, reported that both pastors and imams, particularly in rural areas, supported specific candidates in public religious messages.

[11] Some Catholic and Protestant health care facilities do exist in Francophone Africa, but not in close partnership with the state.

[12] Some bilateral donors also influenced this decision (Interview 13).

[13] While countries with larger populations such as South Africa tend to have more ANERELA+ members than smaller countries such as Malawi, in terms of the percentage of their country's total population, smaller countries are more highly represented in the organization.

[14] Every year, Freedom House measures a country's political rights (e.g., right to compete for office) and its civil rights (e.g., freedom of association and freedom of the press). It classifies countries on a scale of 1-7, with 1-2.5 being "free," 3-5 being "partly free," and 5.5-7 being "not free" (Freedom House 2009).

[15] There are at least two reasons that churches in Uganda did not act strongly against Museveni's rule for many years. First, the regime has permitted a relatively open civil society and free media. Second, Uganda's past conflicts along religious, regional, and ethnic lines may have prevented churches from promoting pluralism and challenging one-party politics (Freston 2001).

[16] This trend is also apparent in Angola and Congo-Brazzaville.

5
The Diverse Influences of Global Connections

AIDS in Africa hit the global agenda with the new millennium. Organizations of people living with HIV/AIDS, such as the Treatment Action Campaign in South Africa and ACT UP chapters in the United States and Western Europe, demanded greater global AIDS treatment access in their protests against pharmaceutical companies and Western governments. Advocacy movements, such as the One Campaign and Health Global Access Project (Health GAP), attracted the attention of the media, policymakers, and citizens (Smith and Siplon 2006).[1] They called for more money for the global AIDS pandemic and, once industrialized countries promised money, they held them to account for their financial pledges. AIDS mobilization stretched beyond the global and national levels to the grassroots. In the United States, for example, church congregations and university student organizations sponsored countless AIDS-awareness days, sent church members on mission trips to work with African AIDS orphans, and raised millions for African community AIDS projects.

All of this activity generated impressive outcomes: Between 1998 and 2008, global funding for AIDS increased from $160 million to $7.7 billion (UNAIDS 2008b). New initiatives emerged, including the World Bank's Multi-Country AIDS Program (MAP Initiative), the Global Fund, and PEPFAR in 2000, 2002 and 2003, respectively. With the assistance of the World Bank and UNAIDS, African governments began to establish formal AIDS policy-making institutions and to build the organizational capacity to manage the huge sums of funding they began to receive (Putzel 2004; Haven 2005; Patterson 2006; Epstein 2007).

The previous two chapters have shown how resources within the church—biblical frameworks, organizational structures, and pastoral leadership—and church-state relations influence church AIDS activities. My purpose in this chapter is to show how African churches are situated within a complex web of international AIDS activities which also condition church responses to the pandemic. African institutions are often portrayed as either victims of global forces beyond their control or as instrumental opportunists that use public and private means to gain donor resources (Chabal and Daloz 1999; Myandawire and Souldo 1999). This chapter provides nuance to those images. First, it analyzes the complicated ways that churches are both influenced by external forces and act independently in their dealings with global actors. To do so, I examine the relationships between churches and donors, defining donors broadly to include both bilateral and multilateral AIDS programs. Second, the chapter moves beyond the assertion that it was solely donor money that caused churches to act on AIDS. I make this second point through an analysis of how ideals that were present in African churches, global ecumenical organizations, and personal networks influenced the initiation and/or implementation of church AIDS activities. Because most global attention to AIDS occurred after 2000, international forces had the greatest effect on more recent church activities. However, as the cases below illustrate, external forces (often in tandem with local church agency) shaped the scope of church actions in different ways.

The chapter's divisions mirror its two broad objectives. In the first major section, I analyze how donor programs influenced church AIDS activities, situating church agency along a continuum from low to high. At the low end of the spectrum, churches appear relatively powerless; they react to donor money and have limited say on program priorities. Most churches fall in the middle of this continuum, and they use donor funds to support their priorities or to empower themselves in AIDS politics. At the high end of the spectrum, a few churches have challenged the AIDS regime, or the structures, norms, and beliefs which undergird donors' work. These churches exhibit autonomy from donors, although not necessarily from other external actors.

The chapter's second section addresses the instrumental view that churches fight AIDS only because they want access to donor money. It asserts that while donor funding may have contributed to AIDS efforts, it is not the only international factor that pushed churches' AIDS actions. African churches participate in ecumenical organizations and global networks, and they have personal interactions with churches and individuals in industrialized countries. The resulting global interactions can be a source of influence, information, and support for AIDS activities.

Donors and Church Agency in AIDS Efforts

Since the late 1980s, donor funds have been crucial in Africa's AIDS fight (Patterson and Cieminis 2005). While donor programs have often been underfunded and sometimes short-lived, their existence illustrates the huge need in Africa for external resources. African countries, with their high poverty rates, poor health care infrastructures, neopatrimonial governance patterns that contribute to mismanagement, and high levels of debt, have limited state resources for AIDS. In some African countries, over 80 percent of AIDS funding comes from bilateral and multilateral donors (UNAIDS 2008b, 258-260). This fact does not discount the hours of volunteer labor and the compassion that millions of Africans (Christians and non-Christians) have shown to people infected with and affected by HIV/AIDS.

It would be naïve to believe that donors have no influence on the actions that churches take to fight AIDS. For example, PEPFAR's emphasis on ARV treatment, but not food distribution, has meant that the Catholic Church in Zambia has had to cut some food security programs, despite the fact that adequate nutrition is needed for ARVs to effectively combat HIV (Fikansa 2009). Throughout my fieldwork, many respondents complained about the ever-changing focus of donor programs (Interviews 3, 9, 10, 14, 16, 18, 22, 30, 35, 50, 60). One Zambian, for example, said that as soon as a church developed a program around one issue, the donor changed focus: "One year it's prevention of mother-to-child transmission and the next, it's orphans and vulnerable children" (Interview 17). One view of these dynamics is that donors drive the agenda, while African churches are passive victims. The cases below, however, show how African church agency varies with the context. By capitalizing on external connections, churches engage in what Jean-François Bayart (1993) terms extroversion. Being situated in a global context provides African churches (just like the African governments Bayart analyzes) with the ability to cultivate a new resource: "Far from being the victims of their very real vulnerability, [African civil society organizations] exploit, occasionally, skillfully, the resources of dependence" (Bayart 1993, 25-26). Linkages to donors may become a tool by which African churches (or their leaders) increase power and ultimately, challenge those donors' own policies and programs.

Before beginning, it is important to recognize that donor AIDS funds slated for faith-based organizations have primarily gone to Christian groups. The lower HIV prevalence rates in Muslim countries and Western donors' connections with international Christian development organizations such as World Vision or Christian Aid are two reasons for this pattern. In Christian-majority African countries, many churches (particularly the Catholics and mainline Protestants) have well-developed organizational structures and grassroots development initiatives; these arrangements make it easier to work with churches than with Muslim groups (Morgan 2010). African traditional religions are even less likely to access donor funds. They often lack centralizing organizations, and it may be hard to define their constituent members. They also face suspicion from Christians and Muslims and from secular governments, who fear their alleged involvement in questionable practices such as human sacrifice or other illegal actions (Cooper 2006; Bornstein 2005; Ellis and ter Haar 2004). As Chapter 3 showed, these patterns in donor funding may affect how African churches interact with these other religious groups.

Donors and Limited Church Agency: Ghana's Compassion Campaign

In general, Ghana's Compassion Campaign illustrates the pattern of donors determining church actions on AIDS. Donors, particularly USAID and the World Bank MAP Initiative, affected both the relatively early timing of the campaign (2000-2003) and its narrow focus. In terms of the scope of the Compassion Campaign, donors pushed the effort to be narrowly focused on prevention and stigma reduction primarily because they wanted to urge AIDS awareness. When the campaign began, ARV treatment was not widely available in Africa, and Ghana's relatively low HIV prevalence meant that donors would not put much funding into large-scale care and support programs.

In terms of timing, as Ghana approached the new millennium, donors were increasingly concerned that the HIV prevalence in West Africa would become as high as it was in southern Africa. Donors pushed Ghana to address the disease before the HIV prevalence reached 5 percent in the general population. This concern was reflected in an uptake in funding. In 2001, Ghana received a $25 million loan from the MAP Initiative to establish the Ghana AIDS Commission and district AIDS councils and to design its multi-sectoral AIDS strategy. As the country's largest bilateral donor, USAID provided $20 million specifically for AIDS in 2002; this amount was over one-third of the total amount of aid that the American agency provided to Ghana in that one year (USAID 2008; Haven and Patterson 2007). USAID contracted with Johns Hopkins University to design an AIDS awareness campaign, part of which became the Compassion Campaign (Interviews 26, 50). Donor funding was crucial for training pastors and lay leaders and for airing mass media messages between 2000 and 2003.

Once the three-year campaign was over, and once it became apparent that Ghana's HIV prevalence level was not rapidly increasing, there was less donor interest in AIDS awareness efforts targeting the general population, such as the Compassion Campaign. USAID shifted the focus of its AIDS programs to populations most at risk for HIV infection, particularly men who have sex with men and commercial sex workers. By 2008, USAID had de-emphasized AIDS and heightened attention to malaria; its AIDS spending dropped to $6.8 million (USAID 2008; Interview 40). Global Fund grants replaced USAID money as the biggest source of donor AIDS funds, and the vast majority of the $63 million in the country's 2003 and 2006 grants was slated for scaled-up ARV treatment and increased HIV testing (Global Fund 2003a, 2006a, 2008a; UNAIDS 2008a). Concerns about most-at-risk populations were further reflected in the country's successful proposal to the Global Fund in 2009: this grant provides roughly $48 million for condom distribution, HIV testing, and AIDS education programs (Global Fund 2010b).

The dynamics of the Compassion Campaign illustrate how donors can shape African church AIDS activities and, at times, limit the agency of churches in these relationships. Four general statements emerge about these dynamics. First, when donors had an interest in AIDS, churches responded and developed the Compassion Campaign. While it appears that churches were just trying to access funds, the second portion of this chapter nuances that assertion. More broadly, it is possible to see that African churches were affected by donors' demands for the campaign.

Second, when donors shifted their priorities to malaria and AIDS funding decreased, church AIDS programs declined. It is possible to see churches as either strong or weak players in the context of the decrease in funding. The churches-as-strong-agents viewpoint asserts that churches were responding to the epidemic's dynamic and the issue's saliency. Despite donors' fears, the country did not experience an HIV prevalence explosion between 2000 and 2008; in fact, the official HIV prevalence dropped from 3.3 percent in 2003 to 1.9 percent in 2007 (UNAIDS 2008a). Over time church members, like the general population, did not view AIDS to be salient. Few Ghanaians reported knowing someone with AIDS (Afrobarometer 2004). As one pastor said: "If I went to church on Sunday and said I was going to preach on AIDS, the congregants would just say, 'Pastor, what do you have to tell us that is new? We have heard it all before'" (Interview 30).

On the other hand, the churches-as-weak-players perspective points to church leaders who wanted to emphasize AIDS but no longer had donor resources to do so.[2] These church actors felt that donors did not want to support the hard programming needed to further lower the country's HIV prevalence. For example, one church official complained that donors would not support AIDS training in theological schools or seminaries (Interview 30). The low level of funding meant churches that were doing grassroots HIV awareness and stigma reduction programs had very low-key efforts; there were no flashy TV ads or billboards. This approach was often under-funded and led citizens to believe that churches were doing nothing on AIDS (Interviews 26, 35).

Third, donors' goal of targeting most-at-risk groups affected churches. Here churches seemed to have limited agency in shaping this donor priority, except in their implicit decision to not participate in this policy initiative. The move to work with commercial sex workers and men who have sex with men made most churches uncomfortable. Some church organizations, such as the Ghana Evangelical Women's Organization, have tried to work with commercial sex workers, but this is difficult. One church leader explained the challenges of these programs:

> When we started working with commercial sex workers, people in the churches said, 'You are not serious, are you? Why are you doing this? You are normal people, but they are not.' Everyone said that the commercial sex workers just want to give the church pastor AIDS. And some of the commercial sex workers thought that the Reverend just wanted to give them AIDS. (Interview 51)

Similarly, because homosexuality is illegal in Ghana, men who have sex with men are not easy to identify for AIDS programs. Only a handful of church leaders have sought to work with this population and "that has not been a popular thing in those congregations" (Interview 30).

USAID's new prevention focus, reinforced through the country's Global Fund grant in 2009, led one interviewee to argue that AIDS policy was dictated by Westerners who do not understand Ghanaian society. The informant continued that Ghana was being "punished" for successfully bringing down its HIV prevalence: "To keep the rate down, though, we need continuous funds for education and behavior change for the broad population" (Interview 27). Another Ghanaian complained that the new focus on most-at-risk populations leads to the idea that only "deviant others" get AIDS (Interview 36). In contrast to the stated intention of the Compassion Campaign, these recent efforts may reinforce the belief that only people outside the church have AIDS.

Fourth, donors' attention to HIV testing has brought new church actors into AIDS work; in doing so, this funding may empower those religious agents. The rate of HIV testing among Ghanaians has been relatively low, because of the stigma and the belief that "only others" get AIDS (Oppong and Agyei-Mensah 2004). While 10 percent of people globally knew their HIV status in 2008, only 8 percent of Ghanaians did. There is concern that if people do not know their HIV status, they will continue to engage in risky sexual practices.[3] Ghana's 2008 Demographic and Health Survey may illustrate this trend: the average age for sexual debut for women was 17 years in 2008, down from 18.3 years in 2003. For men, the decline was from 20 years to 19 years (Interview 34). HIV testing may also help combat Ghana's low rate of ARV uptake; as of 2007, only 15 percent of HIV-positive Ghanaians who needed ARV treatment had access to it, primarily because of low testing rates. In 2008, the Ghana AIDS Commission (with funds from multilateral and bilateral donors) set the ambitious agenda of testing 55,000 people (*Daily Graphic*, November 18, 2008; UNAIDS 2008a).

To meet this HIV testing goal, the Ghana AIDS Commission gave a grant in 2008 to Word Miracle Church, a neo-Pentecostal congregation with several thousand members, to establish a voluntary counseling and testing center in Accra. Working through a mega-church that is popular with urban young people signaled the government's awareness of the need to reach out to as many Ghanaians as possible in its AIDS programs. The action also illustrated that some of these New Independent churches have modified their views on AIDS, no longer viewing the disease merely as a curse from God (Interviews 27, 49). But while bringing new actors into the AIDS fight is crucial, and increases those churches' investment in the issue, one could ask if this incorporation is at the expense of other organizations. Donors such as the Global Fund and PEPFAR need to show results, a fact that pushed their national-level partners to try to reach as many individuals as possible in AIDS programming. For Ghana, this has meant working with large churches in urban centers, instead of smaller churches in rural areas (Interviews 35, 46). It also meant that some of the major players in the Compassion Campaign—Catholics and mainline Protestants—were left out of this HIV testing initiative.

Donor Connections Increase Church Agency and Power

Unlike the case of relatively limited church agency in the Compassion Campaign, the next cases illustrate how some churches have used donor money to reinforce their priorities, to expand their programs, and to augment their power vis-à-vis the state (Epstein 2007; Blumenthal 2009; FBO Roundtable 2009). First, donors may empower churches when their objectives overlap with the church recipient's objectives. PEPFAR's restrictions in its HIV prevention programs illustrate this pattern and they help explain the narrow, recent efforts of churches such as the Makerere Community Church. To see this effect, it is helpful to know more about PEPFAR. The American policy resulted from the growing awareness about AIDS among American evangelical Christians, a crucial Republican voting bloc in the 2000 election (Guth et al. 2006). By 2003, faith-based organizations like Samaritan's Purse and World Vision had mobilized American evangelical Christians to support AIDS programs in Africa. In combination with the public efforts of Republican Senators like Jesse Helms and Bill Frist, a Republican-controlled Congress passed PEPFAR, a program which allocated most of its $15 billion between 2003 and 2008 to fifteen focus countries. (Twelve of the fifteen were in sub-Saharan Africa.) To win the support of Republicans in Congress who often have been skeptical of foreign aid, the legislation needed to be results oriented, to allocate some money directly to faith-based groups, and to de-emphasize condoms. As outlined in Chapter 1, the 2003 law appropriated 20 percent of funding to HIV prevention; 55 percent to ARV treatment; 15 percent to programs that give care and support to people living with HIV/AIDS; and 10 percent to projects for orphans and vulnerable children. The PEPFAR legislation also required that one-third of a recipient country's HIV prevention funding be allocated to abstinence and fidelity programs. The 2008 PEPFAR reauthorization gives countries more flexibility on prevention, but requires them to report to congress if they do not spend half of the prevention funds on abstinence and fidelity programs (*Kaiser Daily HIV/AIDS Report*, July 17, 2008; Patterson 2006).

Because many African churches were uncomfortable with condoms (Illife 2006), the PEPFAR abstinence and fidelity spending requirement presented a new opportunity structure, or a moment in which churches could mobilize in support of narrowly focused HIV prevention priorities. For a few churches, PEPFAR money meant they could scale up already existing abstinence and fidelity programs. For the large number of churches without prior HIV prevention programs, PEPFAR funds meant they could rapidly develop such initiatives (Christiansen 2009). Helen Epstein writes about Ugandan pastors, "After ... PEPFAR [was introduced], a number of the local evangelical preachers began to get excited . . . and get involved in AIDS very rapidly" (cited in Blumenthal 2009). In these cases, churches were not acting solely as *agents of donors*, but as actors that used the new opportunity structure presented by PEPFAR to meet their own objectives. PEPFAR contributed to these more recent church AIDS efforts.

A second pattern is that donors may enable churches to expand already existing programs. Because donor money has come after these programs were established, it does not directly affect their timing or scope. The Kamwokya Christian Caring Community, a Catholic organization in Kampala, provides an example. The church began its AIDS programs in 1987, before donors were paying much attention to AIDS in Africa. Sister Miriam Duggan, an Irish nun working in medical missions, urged these actions, a fact that reinforces Chapter 3's point about leadership and AIDS program initiation. By the mid-1990s, the church had projects in support, care, HIV prevention, stigma reduction, and treatment of opportunistic infections. PEPFAR funding funneled through international faith-based organizations such as Catholic Relief Services, in addition to individual donations from other faith-based groups, enabled them to scale up these projects, develop a child advocacy program, and provide ARV treatment to approximately 7,000 in the community. It seemed these efforts further increased the church's independence in the public realm, and it began to engage more intentionally in lobbying the national government on AIDS and development issues.[4]

The tendency of some donors to funnel money to civil society groups instead of the state also may increase the power of churches. The case of CHAZ and the Global Fund illustrates this point. As with the Kamwokya Christian Caring Community, CHAZ had AIDS efforts in prevention, treatment of opportunistic infections, stigma reduction, and care before 2000. Donor money did not determine the scope or timing of CHAZ efforts, although external funds did enable the expansion of AIDS activities, particularly ARV distribution (CHAZ 2005, 2009). As Chapter 4 illustrated, faith-based groups must be represented on a country's CCM and some, such as CHAZ, have become principal recipients of grants. As Table 5.1 illustrates, CHAZ received almost $70 million directly from the Global Fund in two rounds of grants.[5]

Table 5.1 Global Fund Allocations for Zambia (US dollars)

Year and Funding Round	Principal Recipients	Amount Requested (for all recipients in round)	Amount Approved (over 5 years)	Amount Dispersed (over 5 years)
2003 (1)	Ministry of Health	92,847,000	40,884,928	35,757,291
	Ministry of Finance		6,395,758	3,057,134
	Churches Health Association of Zambia (CHAZ)		22,840,611	22,840,611
	Zambia National AIDS Network (ZNAN)		20,204,481	20,204,481
2005 (4)	Ministry of Health	263,318,738	116,128,561	29,665,720
	Ministry of Finance		15,766,759	7,382,073
	Churches Health Association of Zambia (CHAZ)		71,400,023	46,077,638
	Zambia National AIDS Network (ZNAN)		33,023,395	14,575,239
2008 (8)	To be determined	307,273,165	144,079,863	
Total Dispersed				**179,560,187**

Source: Global Fund 2003b, 2005, 2008b.

The health association's allocation was one-third of the total amount that Zambia got from the Global Fund in those two rounds. In contrast to alleged funding mismanagement in some Zambian ministries, CHAZ has exhibited transparency and accountability in grant management and has received much of its approved grant money (*BBC News*, July 16, 2009; *Zambian Post*, June 16, 2010).[6]

The health association's wide reach and its relations with government through the memorandum of understanding meant it always had a voice in health care policy. However, some interviewees argued that resources from the Global Fund and PEPFAR have given CHAZ greater power in its interactions with the government (Interviews 6, 13). As a result, CHAZ successfully advocated to eliminate user fees at health facilities in 2006 and to provide free ARVs in 2005 (Interviews 13, 15). Since most of its external resources come from the Global Fund, not a bilateral donor, CHAZ may have had greater flexibility when donors changed AIDS program priorities. For example, when some Western donors wanted to give CHAZ money to do HIV prevention efforts among men who have sex with men, CHAZ refused the funding (FBO Roundtable 2009). As a CCM member, CHAZ has had autonomy in designing programs to meet its constituency's needs.

The heightened church agency that can result from donor funds may lead to a third trend, changes in church-state relations. As Chapter 4 argued, church-state relations in Africa are fluid; churches invade the public square to advocate for policies or particular values while the state incorporates religious symbols and rhetoric to justify its actions. Donor resources add an additional element to this relationship, particularly on a continent where resources are in short supply and neopatrimonial state practices make access to resources important. Most African states do not have the resources to tackle AIDS, and specifically to provide ARVs. While donors work with the state to develop strategic AIDS plans or to set up AIDS institutions, the state only receives a portion of donor AIDS money. PEPFAR prime partners, for example, are often international nongovernmental organizations and American universities. And while 60 percent of Global Fund grant money goes to government ministries, 29 percent goes to faith-based organizations, multilateral donors (such as UNICEF), and international and national-level nongovernmental groups (Global Fund 2007).[7] As Chapter 4 showed, faith-based groups in Zambia, Zimbabwe, and Ethiopia have received large sums of Global Fund money.

A paradox emerges. Elected African governments face pressure from civil society and the media to show that they are addressing issues important in citizens' lives. Yet, governments do not get most of the external funding needed to play this role. Instead, international and local nongovernmental organizations and faith-based organizations, which are not accountable to African citizens in the ways that governments theoretically are, receive resources. These international agencies fund local partners, who often have more accountability to the donor than they do to their own members (Patterson 2006; Šehović 2010). This dynamic may lead Africans to discount their rights and responsibilities as citizens in the social contract with the state (Interview 61).

Zambia illustrates this accountability problem. In 2007, the NAC, the government institution for AIDS policy-making and implementation which is supposed to coordinate the country's AIDS programs and make sure they meet the Strategic Framework's objectives, had a budget of only $5 million. In contrast, CHAZ and the Zambian National AIDS Network received $70 million and $53 million respectively from the Global Fund. It was estimated that non-state actors in Zambia receive roughly $370 to $400 million annually for AIDS, including funding from bilateral donors and the Global Fund. One informant explained that it is difficult for the government to coordinate all of the AIDS activities in the country; it may not even know what is going on with all of the organizations working on AIDS. The interviewee continued: "The NAC with its small amount of money just doesn't stand a chance. . . . How then can government be held accountable for the country's AIDS situation" (Interview 13)?

While states may value churches' AIDS efforts, donor-funded church activities point to the state's inadequacy. Through their activities, the churches are playing (whether intentionally or not) a subversive role; they are helping to underline the state's limitations and contribute to its lack of legitimacy. Citizens will be much less likely to criticize churches than state officials for limited AIDS efforts, a fact which further bolsters church power in this dynamic. One Ghanaian interviewee explained this scenario in the context of the Compassion Campaign:

> There was some suspicion from people [on the Compassion Campaign] that there was some competition with the GAC [Ghana AIDS Commission] over the campaign. [This feeling] that we [on the Campaign] did our thing and then you'd look on TV and they'd [GAC] have some new ad that looked a lot like our efforts. Some of us felt this way, that there was a bit of tension or competition, because they were supposed to be the ones taking up the mantle of AIDS at that point [but they weren't]. (Interview 50)

As donor funds help churches increase their autonomy and power vis-à-vis the state, these churches' internal accountability and their relations with other churches may be affected. Donor money may exacerbate a centralizing tendency in some churches and enable the pastor to set program priorities with donors without the input of congregants. While power centralization can emerge without donor money, the benefits of controlling decisions increase when money is involved. Since many African churches lack strong institutions to provide checks on pastoral power, particularly Pentecostal churches that are started by one individual (Kalu 2008), there is greater possibility for external funding to foster power centralization. Thus, another paradox emerges: churches need entrepreneurial leaders to help them access donor funds, but such leaders may then use resources to increase their own status, garner more media attention, and foster their own agendas. The pastor's popularity helps the church increase its membership. Popular pastors who lead large churches may more easily access donor resources because donors want to reach large numbers of people with their messages and programs. This cycle does not necessitate greater accountability within the church.

As pastors increase in power and resources, they may compete with one another for funds, members, and prestige (Bodewes 2009; Gusman 2009). Events in 2009 among Ugandan Pentecostal pastors illustrate this negative outcome. Martin Ssempa and Simon Male, pastor of the Arise and Shine Ministries in Kampala, accused another Pentecostal pastor, Robert Kayanja of Kampala's Miracle Centre Church, of sodomizing boys in his congregation after the boys told Ssempa and Male about their alleged experiences. The police questioned all three pastors, and eventually found the allegations to be "baseless." After the boy who had accused Kayanja explained that he had been "used by some pastors" to destroy Kayanja's reputation and ministry, the head of police investigations attacked the credibility of the church leaders (*New Vision*, May 17, 2009). The intense nature of the conflict demonstrates that a rivalry among Pentecostal pastors in Uganda has developed, as churches compete for members and funds, primarily from American congregations (*New Vision*, May 18, 2009). Since Pentecostals often stress morality and holy living, accusations of sexual impropriety could be particularly damaging to a pastor's reputation. Absent in this example are strong institutions to hold these leaders accountable and temper their public actions. Without such structures, inter-church competition may urge pastors to play "dirty politics." To be clear, it is not that donor funds caused these actions; but they contribute to a larger dynamic of increased power among donor recipients. More in-depth case studies are needed to fully appreciate the ways donor resources have shaped the internal politics of churches.

Donors, Independent Church Agents, and Challenges to the AIDS Regime

In some cases, churches act as agents that independently challenge the AIDS regime. Some of these churches have never received donor funds or participated in donor-designed AIDS efforts, but others have. There may be a reciprocal relationship between these churches' independence from donors and donor-provided resources: a church may have a strong voice on AIDS, a fact which makes donors attracted to it. With donor funding, the church may gain greater agency in AIDS politics. To be clear, my focus is church independence from donors, not necessarily from Western (primarily American) congregations. Ties to Western congregations may increase the ability of African churches to challenge the AIDS regime. It is difficult to determine relations of power and dependence in these ad hoc cross-national relationships. On the one hand, journalists report that American evangelical churches increasingly support the operating budgets and building funds of African churches (Gorter 2006; Kaoma 2010). On the other hand, African church leaders fiercely defend their independent positions (Englund 2003). It is also unclear to what extent Western church money may "create a form of clientelism, with the expectation that the recipients toe an ideological line" (Kaoma 2010, 6). It does seem though that these resources give some pastors the freedom to speak out against the major tenets of the donor-related AIDS regime.

To better understand these churches' backlash, it is necessary to provide some history. The AIDS regime is rooted in the biomedical approach to AIDS and a liberal understanding of human rights. The regime recognizes well-established scientific facts about the virus, its modes of transmission, and the role of ARVs in limiting viral load (Youde 2007; Iliffe 2006; Seidel 1993). The reciprocal relationship between human rights and AIDS is also emphasized. Jonathan Mann (1999) argued that AIDS proliferates in conditions where human rights violations (such as gender-based violence and inadequate access to food and medical care) are prevalent. In turn, HIV infection leads to human rights violations, with stigma and discrimination negatively impacting people infected with or affected by HIV/AIDS (Csete 2007).

Some state and non-state actors have criticized the AIDS regime because of its roots in Western liberalism, a philosophy which portrays individuals as autonomous actors whose identity does not derive from the community or from a supreme power such as a deity. Liberals assert that individuals with rights exist prior to the formation of a community; people established the community because it protects their personal interests, not out of a shared identity or common goal. The assumption is that individuals have rights and the power to make autonomous decisions (Marshall 1964).

The biomedical and liberal roots of the AIDS regime led donor programs to focus on technical means to decrease HIV transmission. Examples include condom awareness and distribution programs, HIV prevention efforts among most-at-risk groups, HIV testing for pregnant women, and the provision of clean needles for intravenous drug users (Iliffe 2006, 90). HIV prevention programs have often assumed that if individuals have adequate information, autonomy, and the means (such as condoms) to protect themselves from HIV infection, they will rationally choose to do so. Further, the liberal, technical approach to AIDS takes no stand on the moral questions surrounding AIDS. For example, the regime does not criticize commercial sex workers, but seeks to protect them from HIV infection through condom distribution and programs to teach them to negotiate condom use with clients (UNAIDS 2009a; Iliffe 2006).

The establishment of UNAIDS in 1996 helped entrench the AIDS regime. When AIDS emerged in the 1980s, the United Nations developed the Global Programme on AIDS within the World Health Organization. Narrowly focused, the program worked with health ministries to control the epidemic. In contrast, UNAIDS has a broader and more political mandate. It gathers surveillance data on the pandemic, coordinates AIDS efforts among ten UN agencies, publicizes best practices in the AIDS fight, and provides technical assistance to governments for building institutional capital, mobilizing civil society, and organizing awareness campaigns (Patterson and Cieminis 2005).[8] UNAIDS advocates for the disease and the people it affects. The program's first director Peter Piot, who served from 1996 until the end of 2008, built global support to address AIDS, successfully lobbied for huge increases in AIDS funding, and entrenched the biomedical and liberal approach into UNAIDS best practices.

Not only churches have challenged the biomedical and liberal approaches of the AIDS regime. Former South African president Thabo Mbeki questioned the scientific link between HIV and AIDS in 2000. Mbeki's health minister Manto Tshabalala-Msimang maintained that ARVs lacked efficacy, and she urged South Africans to combat HIV with vitamins, nutrition, and even garlic (Patterson 2006). In *The Invisible Cure*, Helen Epstein (2007) questions some aspects of the regime, particularly the idea that individuals can act autonomously to prevent HIV infection. Epstein argues that Uganda brought down its HIV rate through the use of communal pressures that led people to limit risky behavior such as concurrent sexual partners. She situates AIDS in a communal context and asserts that HIV prevention programs that target most-at-risk groups or distribute condoms make the community believe AIDS is a disease that only "others" get. Anthony Simpson's study of highly educated Zambian men who engage in risky sexual relations also challenges the liberal assumption that if given information, people will act rationally to protect themselves from HIV transmission (Simpson 2009).

For churches, their criticisms follow four lines: (1) the regime's emphasis on biomedical healing over spiritual healing; (2) the regime's unwillingness to appreciate African culture while ignoring negative Western influences on Africa; (3) the regime's liberal emphasis on individual identity over communal identity; and (4) the regime's focus on the technical solution of condom distribution over programs that stress sexual abstinence and fidelity. First, a minority of churches that have engaged in spiritual healing reject the biomedical approach. They have urged their HIV-positive members to stop taking their ARVs, to attend special healing ceremonies or camps, and to pray steadfastly (Dilger 2007; Kwansa 2009). These churches illustrate church agency, even though they have not received donor funding. Their actions also present a large health risk to church members who quit taking their ARVs.

There are other churches with a less extreme approach to ARVs: they do not discourage ARV use but remain suspicious of the drugs. Some church leaders fear that AIDS treatment will enable HIV-positive people to be sexually irresponsible. Others are concerned that the regime's recent drive to increase ARV access in Africa has meant less attention is given to care, support, and prevention activities. A Malawian pastor demonstrates suspicion of both the AIDS regime and people living with HIV/AIDS: "ARVs are being pushed by medical and social activists just as the condom was being pushed. The danger here is that the healthier the infected people look, the more likely they would [be to] infect others should they be promiscuous" (Kalipeni, Muula, and Liwewe 2009). These leaders' lack of enthusiasm about ARVs presents challenges to successful ARV adherence and expanded ARV uptake in Africa (Msoka 2009).

A second church criticism of the AIDS regime is that because it focuses on biomedical solutions, it ignores the negative influences of Western culture on the sexual behavior of African youth. African churches with this criticism reflect the public opinion of their countries. In a 2010 survey, for example, 67 percent of Zambians, 73 percent of Ugandans, and 74 percent of Ghanaians said they believed that Western movies and music hurt morality (Pew Forum 2010).[9] These church leaders argue that the AIDS regime discounts the positive aspects of African society, such as family obligations or traditional norms against sex before marriage (*BBC News*, May 10, 2003). In the era of globalization, urban youth are exposed to Western media, movies, and music, some of which approach sexual relations from a perspective of liberal autonomy. These churches are reacting to a context where urban migration, income inequality, and the colonial experience have eroded some of the communal and religious norms that traditionally curtailed sexual behavior (Whiteside 2005).

Third, many churches have been uneasy with the ways the liberal, technical approach to AIDS downplays communal identity and expectations. They argue that AIDS programs must take into account not only the rights of the HIV-positive person, but also the effects of the disease on everyone with whom that person interacts. This communal understanding of AIDS is evident in the issue of pre-marital HIV testing. In the United States, HIV testing is confidential and voluntary; there are only a few conditions (such as military service) under which individuals must be tested and, only in exceptional cases can a health professional reveal a patient's HIV status to his or her partner.[10] In Africa, churches have struggled with HIV testing: Should it be required before a church marriage (the position of some Pentecostals) or should it be recommended (the position of some mainline Protestants)? Beyond the individual, who, if anyone, should have access to test results? The response from a Ghanaian informant is fairly typical. The interviewee explained that before a couple gets married, the pastor should insist on couples testing, or a process in which both partners are counseled and tested at the same time and results shared. If one partner tests positive, this information should not be kept from the families of both partners; they should be informed because AIDS will eventually affect the families. That is, family members may have to care for a sick daughter or son, support surviving grandchildren, or pay medical expenses (Interview 43). For the informant, failure to disclose one's HIV status to family members and get their support for the marriage could have negative ramifications beyond the two individuals. Communal responsibility trumps the AIDS regime's focus on individual rights.

The church backlash against the AIDS regime is the most evident in the fourth critique: the churches' perception that the regime emphasizes condom use over abstinence and fidelity. To be clear, church positions on condoms vary widely. The official Catholic Church position forbids condom use, even for sero-discordant, married couples. In reality, some Catholic priests and nuns have spoken in favor of condom use in marriage, while others have privately supported condoms for non-married individuals (*Associated Press*, January 19, 2005; Alsan 2006; Interview 41). Most Protestants state that condoms can be used in marriage to prevent sexually transmitted diseases and pregnancy (*UN Integrated Regional Information Networks*, June 1, 2006). Even for churches that do not promote condoms, they might not explicitly admonish them, recognizing that "we [church members] have to be realistic about sexual behavior" (Interviews 16, 54; FBO Roundtable 2009). Churches that oppose condoms argue that condom use gives the individual a feeling of confidence against HIV infection but does not require sexual responsibility in relationships (Green and Ruark 2008).[11] The anti-condom position challenges the liberal idea that individuals may engage in non-coerced, sexual relations with consenting, adult partners as long as they protect themselves and their partners with condoms. African church opposition to condoms has become more vocal as the AIDS regime has become more entrenched.

These four criticisms of the AIDS regime have fostered narrow and recent church AIDS activities. Early and comprehensive approaches to AIDS incorporated some of these criticisms, but also tried to address AIDS more holistically. For example, Catholic opposition to condoms is a narrow focus within the one area of HIV prevention, but Catholic involvement in advocacy, treatment, support, and care demonstrates the church's broader AIDS responses. Churches that narrowly focus on spiritual healing of HIV, for example, reacted to the increased availability of ARVs in Africa after 2003; churches that emphasize HIV prevention programs that concentrate on abstinence and fidelity messages are a reaction to the technical focus on condoms and HIV awareness programs.

Three of the church criticisms of the AIDS regime are exemplified in the AIDS efforts of Pastor Ssempa and the Makerere Community Church. As Chapter 2 described, the church is not divorced from the AIDS regime: it has received funding from PEPFAR and the Global Fund. Additionally, Chapter 3 illustrated that some African churches have relationships with American evangelical churches. These ties seemed to be strongest between 2002 and 2008, and some of these relationships extended beyond work on the AIDS issue. In 2004, Ssempa told the *New Republic* that "ninety-nine percent of our support comes from the U.S." When the pastor needed to buy land in Kampala, he raised $60,000 from a single church in Columbia, Maryland (Rice 2004). Since then, some American evangelicals have supported his anti-homosexual activities, but others have not (Kaoma 2010; *New York Times*, January 3, 2010; *Newsweek*, December 19, 2009). It would be simplistic to view Ssempa as merely a pawn of Western conservatives. Instead, donor money and external ties seem to have increased the church's agency, and particularly, the independent voice of its pastor against donor programs. This is because his views are coherent with the perspectives of some conservative American evangelical churches.

First, Ssempa faults the AIDS regime for ignoring the negative effects of Western culture on the behavior of African youth. On his website, Ssempa describes how his past lifestyle of girlfriends and parties emulated that of some American performers (see Chapter 3). He then points out that such a lifestyle led his brother to become infected with HIV and eventually, to die of AIDS, and he cautions youth against such a path (Ssempa 2009). Similarly, he speaks about the detrimental effects of the spread to Africa of what he sees as unique Western issues—homosexuality, abortion, prostitution, and pornography. He has led anti-pornography and anti-abortion campaigns and, more recently, he has spoken out against the dangers of what he perceives to be the Western import of homosexuality.

His rhetoric about the moral danger of homosexuality links to his criticism of the AIDS regime (*BBC News*, November 28, 2007; *Monitor*, August 31, 2007). When a Kampala-based study published in the journal *AIDS Behavior* advocated inclusion of homosexual men in Uganda's HIV prevention programs (Kajubi et al. 2008), Ssempa responded, "Previous experience showed us that bringing homosexuals into campaigns against HIV only gives them a chance to propagate their illegal and unnatural acts" (*BBC News*, May 24, 2008). His campaign against homosexuality has included publishing the names of gays and lesbians in the local press, thus placing them in potential physical danger. In one illustration of this risk, in 2008 three Ugandan activists from the gay, lesbian, bisexual, and transgender community were imprisoned after they protested a Ugandan AIDS Commissioner's statement that "meager resources [mean] we cannot direct our programs to [most-at-risk groups such as men who have sex]" (Human Rights Watch 2008). Because Uganda has received large amounts of donor money for AIDS and because Ssempa's anti-homosexual rhetoric has received attention from Western human rights organizations and AIDS activists, the arrests led to greater scrutiny of the country's policies. Global human rights activists began to urge the US Congress to cut PEPFAR funding for Ssempa's HIV prevention programs (Human Rights Watch 2007), and these activities further fueled the pastor's assertion that homosexuals in the West were intent on a gay-rights agenda in Africa (Ssempa 2010).

The situation became more intense in 2009, when the Ugandan Parliament drafted the Anti-Homosexuality Act. The proposed law banned gay organizing and gave the death penalty to homosexuals who had sex with someone underage or while infected with HIV. The bill also made it illegal to "promote, fund, or sponsor" any homosexual practice or activity and made the "failure to disclose" a homosexual an offense punishable with imprisonment. Ssempa supported the legislation (*Independent*, November 10, 2009).

Western governments, global AIDS experts, and several evangelical and mainline churches decried Ugandan church support for the bill, and particularly Ssempa's leadership on the issue (*Observer*, December 13, 2009; *Newsweek*, December 19, 2009). In January 2010, US State Department officials testified in the US House of Representatives about their attempts to dissuade the Ugandan government from passing the law. In February 2010, President Barack Obama condemned the bill (*Reuters*, February 4, 2010). Over 1,400 physicians and public health officials signed a letter that argued the law would stigmatize people living with HIV/AIDS and damage health care provision in Uganda (Center for Global Health Policy 2010a, 2010b). And Pastor Rick Warren and the American evangelical organization WAIT Training severed ties to Ssempa (*Newsweek*, December 19, 2009).[12]

Again, these responses fueled Ssempa's criticism that the West does not understand African society and that the global gay rights movement is a neocolonial influence on the continent. This perspective is particularly apparent in a letter published on Ssempa's website in response to Rick Warren's 2009 statement against the Uganda legislation. In it, Ssempa and other pastors from the Uganda National Pastors Task Force Against Homosexuality present examples of a perceived homosexual assault on the country: increased incidents of homosexual abuse of children and UNICEF's production of a "pro-gay book." The letter chastises Western churches for treating homosexuality with "kid gloves [and] as a minor, private issue" and for allowing homosexuals into positions of social influence, "particularly the church." The letter concludes with demands for a formal apology from Warren for "insulting the people of Africa by your very inappropriate bully use of your church and purpose driven pulpits to coerse [*sic*] us into the 'evil' of Sodomy and Gaymorrah [*sic*]" (Ssempa 2010).

Second, Ssempa's actions reflect the criticism that the AIDS regime focuses on individual rights over the larger communal good. As mentioned above, the AIDS regime has incorporated a human rights perspective that seeks to fight discrimination against people living with or affected by HIV/AIDS. The regime tries to fight stigma by urging government and civil society leaders to disclose their HIV status and by promoting the message that one can live "positively" with HIV. Ssempa has criticized this emphasis on stigma reduction and anti-discrimination, which he terms "politically correct." In 2006, he complained about Botswana's "Miss HIV-Stigma Free" Beauty Contest and lambasted proposals to hold a similar contest in Uganda. To Ssempa, such efforts give AIDS an "attractive, sexy face" and reduce people's perception of risk to an "ugly disease" (*New Vision*, July 29, 2005). More broadly, the pastor dislikes how such efforts assume that individuals act autonomously from the community.

Third, Ssempa has also been critical of the AIDS regime on the condom issue. In 2005, he urged the United Nations to dismiss Stephen Lewis, the UN Special Envoy for HIV/AIDS in Africa, because of what Ssempa termed "his personal agenda of condomising developing nations" (*UN Integrated Regional Information Networks,* September 8, 2005; *BBC News*, September 9, 2004; *Monitor*, October 10, 2005; *BBC News*, August 22, 2007; *New Vision*, March 27, 2008). Ssempa argues that not only does the liberal AIDS regime push condoms, but it also ridicules those who abstain from sex or act responsible in their sexual relationships: "When do they [international organizations] have marriage or abstinence as a World AIDS Day theme" (*UN Integrated Regional Information Networks*, November 3, 2006)? While his anti-condom, pro-abstinence stance is not unusual among African churches, Ssempa's use of parades and rallies to gain media attention certainly is.

The pastor's critiques of the AIDS regime are not without national and global support. Numerous pastors I interviewed said they did not support condoms. Instead, they stressed the need for messages of abstinence before marriage, fidelity, and commitment in relationships in their HIV prevention messages (Interviews 7, 16, 23, 30, 33, 37, 47). Similarly, many African pastors fear a "global gay rights movement" (Interview 61). Global events also provide a context for this perceived threat, as African conservatives and Western liberals in mainline Protestant denominations have argued about homosexuality. In 2008, one-third of the world's Anglican primates boycotted the Anglican Communion conference because of the sanctioning of gay unions and ordination of non-celibate gays and lesbians in some Western churches. Uganda has 23 percent of Africa's Anglicans, second only to Nigeria, with 41 percent (Pew Forum 2008). Ssempa also seems to recognize that some conservative Christians in the United States view Africa as the next battleground in the culture wars over sexual morality and homosexuality (Epstein 2007).

Even though Ssempa's rhetoric and actions are often extreme, donors cannot ignore the broader concerns he raises about sexual morality, communal interests over individualism, and culturally appropriate means to address AIDS for two reasons. First, as Chapter 4 illustrated, pastors are highly trusted and influential, and they have the potential to shape public opinion and individual sexual behavior. For example, after Pentecostal pastors in Mozambique spoke against a condom social marketing campaign entitled *Jeito* ("talent," "style," or "flair" in local Portuguese), their congregants began to link condoms to sexual promiscuity and to view them as a means of HIV *infection*, not HIV prevention (Pfeiffer 2004).[13] Second, because AIDS experts have recognized that more emphasis on HIV prevention is essential to achieve long-term progress against the pandemic, debates over how to urge HIV prevention increase in political significance (Potts et al. 2008). In the future, the dialectic between the AIDS regime and its vocal challengers will affect how, or if, prevention goals are met.

On the other hand, church leaders or congregations that blame or ostracize people living with HIV/AIDS, that denounce the established science on AIDS, or that make extreme statements (such as the Archbishop of Maputo did when he said that HIV-tainted condoms had been sent to Africa to kill people) make it harder for donors to seriously consider their criticisms. These churches may hinder cooperation between all churches, on the one hand, and donors, scientists, AIDS activists, and governments, on the other (*BBC News*, September 27, 2007). In particular, people living with HIV/AIDS may simply view churches to be part of the problem in the AIDS fight, rather than part of the solution (Marshall 2008a; Interviews 19, 39).

To summarize: African churches are not impotent in their dealings with donors, although their leverage in the relationship varies. In some cases, such as the Compassion Campaign, donor money helped initiate church AIDS actions and determined the scope of such activities. At other times, as with CHAZ, donor money empowered the organization to shape policy, although this empowerment then had an effect on church-state relations. Some churches (such as the Makerere Community Church) have gained donor funds but also challenged the broader AIDS institutions. These outcomes mean donors must continue to pay attention to religion in order to limit a backlash against the AIDS regime or to avoid ineffective AIDS campaigns. In turn, religious leaders must refrain from vilifying the regime. As one interviewee noted, the complexity of the pandemic requires greater consultation between secular and religious activists and "honest attempts at listening and compromise" (Interview 61).

Instrumentalism: Is It Only about the Money?

The goal of the last half of this chapter is to build on the prior analysis of African church agency and to investigate the popular perception that African churches developed AIDS programs for the sole purpose of gaining donor money (Epstein 2007; Blumenthal 2009). I do not discount the evidence for the instrumental perspective: African church AIDS efforts rapidly multiplied after the passage of PEPFAR.[14] Some interviewees clearly stated that some churches think that "AIDS is about the money" (Interview 44) or that "AIDS programs are a cash cow" (Interview 50). In reality, the picture is more complicated. Ideals shared among African churches, membership in both formal and informal ecumenical networks, and personal relationships between Western citizens and Africans also drove church AIDS activities.

I will briefly touch on the ways broad ideals have influenced African church AIDS activities. The call for greater social justice found in the Catholic Church since the 1970s influenced an early and broad AIDS response. After Vatican II (1962-1965), the global Catholic Church sought to become more socially relevant. Some Latin American bishops took this charge and advocated for greater mobilization to address unequal economic, political, and social structures in order to foster justice (Vanden and Prevost 2006). One means for doing this was through community organizing and grassroots literacy campaigns. Even though this justice focus affected Catholics in Africa to varying degrees (Longman 2010), it did lead many churches to address AIDS relatively early and to focus on holistic development. This was apparent, for example, in the aforementioned programs of the Kamokya Christian Caring Community.

Additionally, the concept of African church independency, or the autonomy of the African church from Western churches, is a powerful driver of church activities, particularly on the sexual morality questions surrounding AIDS. The Old Mission Churches (Catholics and mainline Protestants) do not want to be perceived as merely extensions of their denominational brethren in the West, and the New Mission Churches do not want to be viewed as puppets of the missionaries that introduced them (Englund 2003). In the AIDS context, independence is particularly evident in the above-detailed opposition to condoms, HIV prevention work with men who have sex with men, or ARV use.

In addition to ideals that may influence church AIDS actions, African church participation in global ecumenical organizations, cross-national networks, and personal relations with Western churches are non-material, international-level drivers of AIDS activities. These three types of relationships have the potential to influence the timing and scope of African church AIDS activities, and through them, African churches may also demonstrate different levels of agency. As was the case with donor funding, however, these types of global relationships (particularly the more institutionalized ones) are more developed for Christians than for Muslims or for people who practice African traditional religions. This means non-Christians are less likely to gain the benefits associated with such global organizations, such as well-developed capacity in fund raising, lobbying governments, and publishing and disseminating information. The lack of such connections may hamper non-Christian AIDS efforts on the continent, particularly in Christian-majority countries.

African Churches and Global Ecumenical Organizations

After African states gained independence in the 1960s and 1970s, many churches increased their participation in global ecumenical bodies. These organizations were initially most important for the Old Mission Protestants (mainlines); by the 1970s, New Mission Protestants (the faith missions, Wesleyans, and some Pentecostals) had increased their participation at the national and global levels. The Old Independents, such as the Zionists and *Aladura*, have participated in the international Organization of African Instituted Churches. On the other hand, New Independent churches (neo-Pentecostals and charismatics) have had limited participation in these organizations. In the next two sections, I focus on four of these global ecumenical organizations: the World Council of Churches, the All Africa Conference of Churches, the World Alliance of Reformed Churches, and the World Evangelical Alliance.[15] Each has played a slightly different role in addressing AIDS on the continent, with the World Council of Churches arguably being the largest player. Before I begin, I provide background on these four organizations.

The biggest, most recognized of these is the World Council of Churches, with a membership of almost 350 Protestant churches and denominations in over one hundred countries. Members include churches from all Protestant classifications outlined in Chapter 1, although it has been dominated by the Old Mission churches such as the Presbyterians, Anglicans, and Methodists. Although not a member of the World Council of Churches, the Catholic Church works closely with the Council and sends representatives to all Council meetings (WCC 2009, 2010). Created after World War II to urge cooperation among churches, the World Council of Churches was dominated by churches from

Western countries until the early 1980s, after which African churches became the majority of members (Davies 1983). This majority status enabled African churches to independently drive the organization's agenda. For example, the World Council of Churches established a special fund to support the anti-apartheid movement in South Africa as well as the liberation movements in Angola, Rhodesia, and Mozambique (Welch 2001, 863). The organization also helped to build African church capacity through educational efforts and information sharing. Capacity building efforts resulted from an internal debate over a moratorium on Western missionaries to Africa. (Catholics also had this debate.) While the moratorium never occurred, the discussion forced the World Council of Churches (and its related institution, the All Africa Conference of Churches) to improve leadership training and educational opportunities for African clergy (Mugambi 1996, 9). Despite criticisms that the organization is too bureaucratic and political (*Economist*, February 23, 2008), the Council has provided leadership on the AIDS pandemic.

The second organization, the All Africa Conference of Churches, was formed in 1963, and represents roughly 120 million African Christians (AACC 2008). As with the World Council of Churches, its membership comes from all types of Protestant churches, although leadership has tended to be from the mainline denominations. As a member of the World Council of Churches, it works closely with the global organization, and several of its leaders have gone on to assume high-profile positions within the World Council. By unifying churches, the All Africa Conference of Churches seeks to strengthen the voice of African churches on social and political issues, from human rights violations to health and development issues. It views itself as an agent of social transformation, a prophetic voice to push for solutions to the continent's problems (WCC 2010).

Third, in 1970 the World Alliance of Reformed Churches, an organization of Presbyterian and Reformed churches, formed. Before its 2010 merger with the Reformed Ecumenical Council, it had 218 member churches with more than 76 million members who belonged to the Alliance because they saw it as an instrument of common witness and service; 121 of its member churches also belonged to the World Council of Churches. The Alliance's goal was to facilitate global ecumenism, and many members of the Alliance were among the pioneers of the World Council of Churches. One of the central ways the Alliance played this leadership role was through intense study of issues and the release of theological statements on topics such as economic injustice, ecological destruction, apartheid, and the human rights of homosexual persons (WARC 2009). For example, in 1982 it explicitly stated that apartheid was a sin and its moral and theological justification was heresy (WCC 2010).

The fourth organization is the World Evangelical Alliance, an organization formed in 1951 but with roots in the Second Great Awakening that occurred in England in the 1840s. The World Evangelical Alliance gained church members rapidly throughout Africa and Asia during the 1970s and 1980s, as evangelical fervor led Western missionaries (primarily Americans) to spread the Gospel globally and begin new churches. This evangelism caused a negative reaction among African mainlines and Catholics. They challenged these missionaries' tendency to link the Gospel to an anti-communist ideological agenda and to portray liberation movements in South Africa, Namibia, and Rhodesia as "ungodly and communist" while tacitly supporting the racist regimes in those countries (Mugambi 1996, 7). The African mainlines and Catholics also criticized the American evangelicals' "utopian" theology, with its focus on morality and individual salvation instead of social justice, long-term development, and human rights (Gifford 1992). After the Cold War, the World Evangelical Alliance grew more, reflecting the spread of Pentecostalism and the increased involvement of the spirit-filled churches on social issues. As a result of these factors, by 2009 the World Evangelical Alliance had church members in 128 countries, and it represented over 420 million evangelical Christians globally (WEA 2009).

How have these four ecumenical organizations been involved on AIDS? With the end of the Cold War, policymakers and the public in Western countries showed little interest in Africa and had limited desire to provide foreign aid to the continent (Lancaster 2000). Ecumenical bodies sought to be relevant to African churches and to rejuvenate interest in the continent throughout industrialized countries. The growing awareness of the AIDS pandemic and its links to poverty and inequality provided such an opportunity, although each of the four organizations approached the issue in a slightly different way. Incorporating a liberationist theology, the World Alliance of Reformed Churches worked from 1997 to 2004 on the Accra Confession. The document emphasized socioeconomic inequalities and the negative effects of globalization for the world's poorest people, and it urged Western church goers to re-evaluate their commitment to the world-wide church community (WARC 2004). The confession placed AIDS in a larger context of unequal global political and economic structures. It did not, however, set a specific strategy for acting on its principles.

The All Africa Conference of Churches had a large role in advocacy, particularly at its general assembly meetings that are held every five years. These well publicized events have enabled the General Secretary to issue pointed statements on the pandemic and the attendees to participate in AIDS awareness campaigns (*Daily Champion*, November 27, 2003; *African Church Information Service*, September 16, 2002; *All Africa News Agency*, March 24, 2000). In addition to this advocacy role, the All Africa Conference of Churches has worked with the World Council of Churches on AIDS activities. The third organization—the World Evangelical Alliance—has focused less on theological critiques or high-level public advocacy, and more on grassroots awareness, particularly among Western congregations. As the next section details, these efforts are evident in the Micah Challenge, a loose network of churches and faith-based organizations from across the world.

The approach of the fourth organization—the World Council of Churches—has combined elements seen in the other three organizations. The World Council of Churches worked closely with the All Africa Conference of Churches to provide a theological critique of economic inequalities and to outline two specific objectives in the AIDS fight: advocacy and capacity building. In terms of advocacy, the World Council of Churches, faith-based organizations such as Tearfund, and Protestant ecumenical councils in several African countries formed the Ecumenical Advocacy Alliance in 2000. The Ecumenical Advocacy Alliance's initial goal was to lobby donor countries and international organizations for increased attention to and funding for AIDS. (Since 2006, the Ecumenical Advocacy Alliance has broadened its agenda to include food security and global fair trade.) At a 2001 meeting in Nairobi, the Ecumenical Advocacy Alliance and the World Council of Churches issued a Plan of Action on AIDS in Africa. The document was crucial for urging African Protestant churches to become more explicit in their AIDS efforts (Kelly 2007; Ndhlovu 2007, 53-54). The Nairobi plan emerged before many national churches had designed official AIDS programs, a fact which demonstrates how ecumenical organizations may be more assertive than national church leaders on policy issues because they do not face direct political, social, or congregational pressures (Interview 2). At the United Nations Special Session on HIV/AIDS in 2001, the World Council of Churches also called for greater cooperation among donors, national governments, and churches to fight AIDS (*African Church Information Service*, July 9, 2001; WCC 2001).

To build church capacity, the World Council of Churches formed the Ecumenical HIV/AIDS Initiative in Africa (EHAIA) in 2002. The initiative provides technical assistance and training for churches and small seed grants for specific AIDS programs (Interview 44). Its goal is to promote "an AIDS-competent church" and it has worked with specialized ecumenical organizations such as ANERELA+ and the Network for African Congregational Theology (EHAIA 2002). The latter, formed in 2000 by southern African pastors and seminary professors, has developed theological curriculum on AIDS and educated pastors and lay leaders about the disease (NETACT n.d.).

How did the relatively institutionalized programs of the World Council of Churches shape African church AIDS efforts? First, it is important to recognize that because of the Council's membership, these efforts had the most influence on mainline Protestant AIDS activities. Catholic churches were only tangentially incorporated into the AIDS efforts of the World Council of Churches, and because Pope John Paul II and national bishops in several African countries had already acted by 2000, the World Council of Churches' activities had limited effect on Catholic AIDS efforts. Similarly, the Council's efforts had little impact on the large, urban neo-Pentecostal churches.

The World Council of Churches' initiatives had varying effects on African churches. In Ghana, they contributed to a relatively early church response to AIDS. Coupled with donor funding, these global ecumenical programs were important for the Compassion Campaign. One interviewee explained:

> Without the African summit [in Nairobi] in 2001, there would have been nothing; the church would have done little. There would have been a real divide between those at the top (at the international level in ecumenical bodies) who were acting, and those down below (at the national and sub-national levels), who were doing nothing (Interview 49).

However, all African churches would have experienced the same level of pressure from the 2001 Plan of Action as the churches in Ghana did. Yet, as Chapter 4 illustrated, church response to AIDS varied widely (Interviews 9, 10, 24).

Why did ecumenical actions matter for Ghanaian churches? A primary reason was that elites in Ghana's mainline churches have a long history of participation in the World Council of Churches, the All Africa Conference of Churches, and the Fellowship of Christian Councils and Churches in West Africa (Gifford 1998). The World Council of Churches EHAIA program located its West Africa office in the Christian Council's Accra office space for several years, helping to cement the ties between the AIDS efforts of the Christian Council and the World Council of Churches. The Compassion Campaign also got support beyond the World Council of Churches when the All Africa Conference of Churches, at that time led by Ghanaian Kwesi Dickson, began its "The Church in Africa Has AIDS" campaign in 2001 (Interview 35). The World Alliance for Reformed Churches, led by a Ghanaian, also issued strong public statements on AIDS (Interview 53). And a Ghanaian, who served as the General Secretary of the Fellowship of Christian Councils and Churches in West Africa, was a crucial founding member of the Ecumenical Advocacy Alliance (Interview 49; WCC 2000).

Relations between Ghanaian church leaders and state and secular civil society groups also meant that the church's desire to address AIDS found reinforcement beyond the church. A crucial figure in the Christian Council, the Fellowship of Christian Councils and Churches in West Africa, and the Ecumenical Advocacy Alliance also had personal links to the Director General of the Ghana AIDS Commission. Major civil society participants who mobilized through the Ghana AIDS Network were linked to the Compassion Campaign through their membership in Ghana's mainline churches. Some of the state and civil society actors involved on AIDS also attended the Legon Interdenominational Church at the University of Ghana, where Kwesi Dickson of the All Africa Conference of Churches had been pastor.

Decision making in African politics and society often revolves around personal networks (Chabal and Daloz 1999). While neopatrimonialism is typically viewed as an obstacle to transparent, efficient, and accountable governance (van de Walle 2001), the Ghana case illustrates that personal ties may help mobilize institutions to act on controversial issues. Global ecumenical efforts were reinforced through the national church hierarchy, with its links to civil society and the state. In conjunction with donor funds, these ties pushed the relatively early action of Ghana's Compassion Campaign. This fact demonstrates that Ghanaian church activities were not merely instrumental reactions to donor money; they were also influenced by historical ecumenical relationships. Far from being victims of these global AIDS initiatives, Ghanaian churches helped to develop them.

In terms of the scope of church AIDS activities, the World Council of Churches AIDS efforts focused narrowly on AIDS awareness and issue advocacy, not the development (and financing) of care, support, prevention, or treatment programs. Because many churches had paid little attention to the disease, a primary objective of global ecumenical efforts was to urge African church members and leaders to recognize that "The church has AIDS" (WCC 2001). A secondary goal was to mobilize Christians in industrialized countries to lobby their governments for resources for AIDS programs, including ARV treatment. As Chapter 2 illustrated, the Compassion Campaign in Ghana met the narrow goal of AIDS awareness and stigma reduction. On the other hand, the narrow focus of the global campaign may have not been sufficient to push churches to adopt more comprehensive, long-term efforts, particularly in low HIV prevalence countries like Ghana where donor priorities shifted over time (Interview 46).

Cross-National Networks

In 2004, three years after the World Council of Churches began its AIDS efforts, the Micah Challenge began.[16] While linked to the World Evangelical Alliance, the challenge receives support from various evangelical bodies such as Scripture Union International and from national-level Micah Challenge campaigns. In the United States, evangelical faith-based organizations such as World Relief and World Vision, and advocacy groups such as Sojourners and Evangelicals for Social Action, participate. The organization works primarily through national-level campaigns, with those in the United States, Canada, Australia, Peru, and India being established in 2005. A sub-component of the challenge is the Micah Network, which includes over 260 Christian relief and development ministries throughout the world (Micah Challenge n.d.). In terms of AIDS, the challenge situates the pandemic in the larger context of the eight United Nations Millennium Development Goals, which aim to reduce poverty, promote gender equality, and combat disease (United Nations 2000).

While African church AIDS efforts may be driven partly by the instrumental goal of accessing donor money, the Micah Challenge's promotion of Christian justice also shaped church AIDS activities, particularly in terms of recent advocacy efforts. The challenge's narrow and recent focus on advocacy has helped to educate African Christians about their national political processes and to host meetings between African elected officials and their constituents (Interviews 24, 61). However, because of its relatively small scale and its establishment after many churches had already begun AIDS efforts, interviewees involved in the challenge did not claim the campaign pushed African churches to initiate AIDS programs (Interview 24).

The campaign raises questions about African church agency in global collaboration. One might argue that the challenge's biggest audience is not Africans, but evangelicals in the West, who have often been skeptical about foreign assistance programs. The campaign seeks to educate Western Christians about AIDS, trade, debt, and hunger in Africa so that these individuals can lobby their governments for anti-poverty policies (Interview 55). At times, it seems that African churches are merely a tool in this education process. For example, in 2007, Zambian pastor Lawrence Temfwe travelled to the United States to talk to Christian colleges and churches and then to Washington, DC to meet with policymakers.[17] One American involved with the Micah Challenge explained the benefits of these visits: "It can be very valuable . . . to bring African leaders to the US to meet with key people in Congress" (Interview 55).

This education process also may entail visits by Western churchgoers to African churches and communities. The number of Americans participating in these "short-term missions" throughout the world has significantly increased, from only a few hundred in the 1960s to nearly a million in 2004 (Gifford 2009, 52). In one example, Micah Challenge member World Vision developed the "Pastors Vision Trips" program that takes leaders from large American evangelical churches to Africa so these pastors can see the negative effects of AIDS and poverty on African Christians (World Vision 2009). According to one official, these visits were crucial for educating American evangelicals about AIDS. Many of the participating pastors then directly lobbied their congressional representatives to pass PEPFAR in 2003 (Interview 54).

It is not always the case that these short-term encounters with African churches have tangible outcomes (Interview 55). Kurt Ver Beek (2006) has investigated the long-term effects of visits to developing countries for their American participants. In his survey of American Christians who went on short-term mission trips to Honduras, he finds that even though many participants claimed the trip made them focus on poverty and development issues after they returned to the United States, only 11 percent demonstrated changes to support these goals. For example, few prayed more for poor people or gave more money to anti-poverty organizations.

Also, these visits may undermine African church agency, particularly if visitors make unreasonable demands or exhibit patronizing attitudes. One interviewee said:

> Sometimes these churches in the US want to go to a particular African country to do a 'work project' or to 'help them.' The [American church] wants to throw a lot of money at the African church, but there is a lot of work involved in getting ready [for such a visit] and sometimes it can really lead to some stressful relationships. It is better

> to have encounters and opportunities that really deepen relationships, and really force North Americans and Africans … to interact in ways that move beyond their own national identities. (Interview 55)

Even though these perceived negative effects may demonstrate a lack of African church agency, the reality is more complicated. Bayart's concept of extroversion (1993), or African actors' use of the continent's poverty and assumed dependence to gain material and nonmaterial benefits, provides another lens through which to interpret African church involvement. These forms of collaboration promote the exchange of information and resources between African and Western churches, a crucial factor not only for policy change in the West, but also for advocacy in Africa (Keck and Sikkink 1998). While it had little direct effect on the AIDS responses of African churches, the Micah Challenge indirectly shaped African church efforts through its mobilization of crucial donor support for African AIDS programs. Furthermore, by providing African church leaders "with a platform into [the US] political process," the Micah Challenge opened avenues for those Africans to tell their own stories and to gain resources on their own terms (Interview 55). It helped bring African representation to global policy efforts on AIDS.

Personal Relationships Between American and African Churches

Globalization has made travel to Africa relatively inexpensive, and, in many cases, it has made rapid communication across countries virtually free. Email, Skype, YouTube, cell phones, Facebook, and web pages all facilitate the ties between churches and individual believers in the United States and Africa. These ties differ from the more institutionalized relationships evident in global ecumenical bodies such as the World Council of Churches or even the more fluid issue-oriented networks such as the Micah Challenge. These contacts are frequently ad hoc, short-lived, and rooted in personal relations; they also lack formal structures, rules, or goals. These relationships have little effect on the timing and scope of African church AIDS efforts. Because many of these associations developed after 2000, they did not influence early AIDS efforts although some may have supported already existing activities. Their fluid nature also limits their long-term impact on the scope of African church AIDS activities.

While I do not deny that personal friendships and shared faith perspectives are crucial aspects of these interactions, it would be naïve to ignore the more material aspects of these ties: African partners need resources and powerful representatives, while Western counterparts (often with resources and political power) want to positively influence the continent. These relationships may allow African churches to access resources without lobbying state bureaucracies or approaching donors who demand in-depth grant proposals and financial reports. For the Western churches, the personal contact enables them to bypass denominational structures or government programs to reach their goals. For example, pastors at several evangelical churches in West Michigan have developed ties to individual African congregations. The Michigan congregation raises money, which is periodically delivered to the African church. Emails, digital photos, cell phone calls, and periodic trips by American church members help keep the cross-national relationship alive.[18]

Again, the extroversion concept sheds light on these ties, as illustrated through the relationship between the DuPage Gloc̲al [*sic*] AIDS Action Network (DGAAN) and the Upendo Village in Nairobi, Kenya. DGAAN started in 2002 with the goal of raising awareness among Chicago-area churches about global and local poverty and the AIDS pandemic. Upendo Village is a project founded by Sister Florence Muia of the Assumption Sisters of Nairobi to provide care, support, and medical treatment to people living with HIV/AIDS. The DGAAN-Upendo Village relationship emerged from friendships between several Chicago-area Franciscans who founded DGAAN and Sister Muia. Sister Muia travels annually to the United States to meet with the group, lobby US lawmakers, raise funds, and speak to Chicago-area churches. As a result of Muia's informative visits, DGAAN has mobilized to lobby US representatives and senators from the Chicago-area on poverty reduction, AIDS, and development programs (DGAAN 2008; Upendo Village 2009).

This cross-national relationship has helped Upendo Village meet some of its goals, particularly in the area of ARV treatment. DGAAN has acted as an advocate for the Kenyan project in the US foreign aid bureaucracy. According to one DGAAN member, after PEPFAR's 2003 passage, some Kenyan clinics were being forced to pay for ARVs distributed through PEPFAR even though the drugs were supposed to be free. When DGAAN members in Chicago heard about the situation from Sister Muia, they contacted then US Representative Henry Hyde, who served as chair of the International Affairs Committee in the House of Representatives and was a PEPFAR proponent. After DGAAN's call to Hyde's office, the ARV co-payments quickly ended and the drugs were provided free to Kenyan clients (Interview 56). The DGAAN-Upendo Village relationship shaped the implementation of donor programming on the ground and clearly brought tangible benefits to HIV-positive Kenyans.

Even with these positive outcomes, the relationship does demonstrate a certain power imbalance. The African church organization depended on the Americans to act as its intermediary to PEPFAR and its Kenyan prime partners.[19] For whatever reason—neopatrimonial politics, donors' unwillingness to listen to host country nationals, corruption, and/or the unwillingness or inability of Upendo Village to advocate directly to PEPFAR administrators in Kenya—the organization turned to DGAAN to lobby from the outside. Yet, such external lobbying does not challenge the national political structures or institutions of foreign assistance programs that act as obstacles in participatory, transparent development processes. Without DGAAN, and its members' relationship with a powerful US representative, the ARV copayments may have continued indefinitely. This assessment does not discount the importance of the DGAAN-Upendo Village tie, but the example raises the question: How do churches that face similar problems but lack a powerful American ally negotiate obstacles?

In summary, the second half of this chapter has moved beyond the instrumental assertion that African churches decided to address AIDS because they were just "chasing donor money" (Interview 41). Pan-African ideals, historical participation in ecumenical organizations, and personal networks across countries also mattered. The World Council of Churches shaped church programs in Ghana, and through the EHAIA project, the Council seeks to build capacity to continue church AIDS programs. Issue-based networks such as the Micah Challenge also play a role, particularly because they directly incorporate African voices into efforts to lobby Western donors to allocate promised funds. Even the more personal networks between American and African churches can bring benefits. Yet, beyond the somewhat unique case of Ghana's Compassion Campaign, cross-national interactions were not the driving force that initially led to African church AIDS activities. Instead, they supported, encouraged, or helped to redefine African church efforts, particularly in the post-2001 period. Stating definitively that these global connections either hamper or promote African church agency is problematic. While material inequality, unrealistic expectations, and patronizing attitudes limit agency, African churches' defense of their independence and their growing position in global Christianity foster it.

Conclusion

This chapter has situated African church AIDS responses in the larger context of international attention to the pandemic after 2000. The huge growth in donor AIDS money and donors' increased willingness to fund faith-based groups provided new opportunities for mobilization among African churches. In a complicated dialectic, churches are both influenced by external forces and act independently in their dealings with global actors. Donor funds may empower churches, and some of those churches have challenged the AIDS regime. African churches have criticized condom distribution, the promotion of ARVs over spiritual healing, AIDS outreach programs for men who have sex with men, and Western cultural influences that allegedly encourage risky sexual behavior. Given churches' influence in Africa, donors must consider these objections.

While donor money is an important driver of activities (particularly in the post-2001 arena), the instrumental view that churches addressed AIDS only because they were searching for money is incomplete. Churches are part of larger networks and global relationships. In the case of Ghana, the World Council of Churches supported the church response to AIDS in conjunction with donor attention. On the other hand, the effects of networks such as the Micah Challenge and personal, ad hoc relationships between American and African churches are less apparent. While some may build African church capacity to negotiate with donors or their own governments, these relations may not challenge the political inequalities that make AIDS policy implementation uneven.

Issues never stay on the global political agenda forever. Here it is important to remember that when AIDS cases first emerged in the 1980s, the disease was widely discussed and donor programs developed. By the mid-1990s, AIDS fell off the global agenda. Similarly, foreign aid programs wax and wane based on a country's strategic interests (Lancaster 2000). One Zambian recognized this problem: "[PEPFAR's] high quality is good, but raises questions about future sustainability, because it is hard to sustain that really high quality once the government is then responsible for funding. What is sustainable then is for PEPFAR to last forever" (Interview 18)! Because PEPFAR, as well as other donor AIDS programs, will most likely *not* last forever, one must ask how prepared African institutions are to continue the AIDS fight. The final chapter examines what AIDS mobilization has taught African churches and how they may apply those lessons to the continent's larger socioeconomic and political development.

[1] The One Campaign was formed in 2004 by eleven anti-poverty organizations (Bread for the World Institute, CARE USA, International Medical Corps, International Rescue Committee, Mercy Corps, Oxfam America, Plan USA, Save the Children, World Concern, World Vision, and Debt AIDS Trade Africa—DATA). Its goal is to mobilize Americans against extreme poverty and preventable global disease (see http://www.one.org). Health GAP was formed in 1999 by the Columbia Mailman School of Public Health, ACT UP New York, ACT UP Philadelphia, Doctors without Borders, the Consumer Project on Technology, Essential Action, AIDS Treatment News, Mobilization Against AIDS International, the International Gay and Lesbian Human Rights Commission, and Search for a Cure (see http://www.healthgap.org).

[2] Ghana's successful Global Fund application in 2009 may change this dynamic. The grant will directly award an international faith-based organization, the Adventist Development and Relief Agency (ADRA), funding for community AIDS education, condom distribution, counseling and testing, and stigma reduction. ADRA will work with local religious partners. Although the grant was awarded after my fieldwork, I question its real ability to empower Ghanaian churches since ADRA is an international organization and since it only received about 10 percent of the $48 million awarded. In contrast, the Ministry of Health will receive over $27 million and the Ghana AIDS Commission, over $13 million (Global Fund 2010b).

[3] Studies show that HIV testing has no positive, population-level effect on HIV prevalence, and does not contribute to a consistent reduction in risk for those who test HIV negative (Potts et al. 2008).

[4] Author observations, visit to Kamwokya Christian Caring Community, Kampala, Uganda, July 7, 2010. More information on the organization is available at http://www.kamccc.org.

[5] CHAZ also has received money from PEPFAR, as both a prime partner and a sub-partner, although the PEPFAR grants are relatively small and some are not reported on the PEPFAR website (PEPFAR 2007).

[6] Grants are given in tranches. If Global Fund auditors do not think a recipient is accountable for grant money, the Board will not authorize the release of all tranches.

[7] The Global Fund does not specify recipients for the other 11 percent of grant money (Global Fund 2007).

[8]The ten agencies are the UN High Commissioner for Refugees, the UN Children's Fund, the World Food Program, the UN Development Program, the UN Population Fund, the UN Office on Drugs and Crime, the International Labor Organization, the UN Educational, Scientific, and Cultural Organization, the World Health Organization, and the World Bank.

[9] Illustrating the often inconsistent nature of public opinion, over 50 percent of respondents in these three countries also said they liked these forms of Western entertainment (Pew Forum 2010).

[10] According to the Kaiser Family Foundation (2009), military personnel, prison inmates, immigrants, blood and organ donors, and newborns in some states are required to take an HIV test. Some states allow a health care professional who has administered an HIV test to a patient and who has reason to believe that the patient will not disclose his or her positive status to a partner, to inform the partner.

[11] Some churches also have challenged the effectiveness of condoms on scientific grounds, arguing that condoms have microscopic holes through which the HIV virus can pass. The World Health Organization has disputed such claims, citing studies that show that correct and consistent condom use among sero-discordant couples reduces the rate of infection to less than 1 percent of couples per year (*Guardian*, October 9, 2003; WHO 2000).

[12] Until January 2010, WAIT Training, an American group which promotes abstinence until marriage helped schedule Ssempa's speaking engagements in the United States. In January 2010, however, WAIT Training broke ties with Ssempa over his anti-homosexual activities. The American organization's website read: "WAIT Training does not affiliate, endorse, associate or partner with anyone seeking to hurt or wound others. Our goals are to impart skills to help all individuals have healthy relationships, to live well, love well and if they choose, to marry well. Recent developments in Uganda and around the world associated with Martin Ssempa have caused us to sever all former associations with him. We have requested he remove all wording on his web site that references our organization." See http://www.waittraining.org.

[13] For over twenty years, social marketing has dominated health education programs in the developing world. The social marketing concept centers on the use of commercial advertising and private sector distribution of health products to promote changes in an individual's behavior. Products are sold at a relatively low price in crucial distribution arenas. Mosquito bed nets, birth control medicines, and condoms are just a few items that have been socially marketed in Africa. Critics have argued that social marketing is ineffective, ignores structural constraints on health-related behavior, and excludes community empowerment and participation in health (Pfeiffer 2004). In recent years, social marketing has become less central, particularly for mosquito bed net campaigns.

[14] Informal conversation with official of Mozambican faith-based organization, Grand Rapids, Michigan, June 4, 2007; informal conversation with official of Kenyan faith-based organization, Grand Rapids, Michigan, October 21, 2009.

[15] In June 2010, the World Alliance of Reformed Churches and the Reformed Ecumenical Council formed the World Communion of Reformed Churches. Because this event occurred as this work was near completion, I focus here on past actions of the World Alliance of Reformed Churches.

[16] The Micah Challenge refers to the biblical challenge presented in Micah 6:8: "And what does the Lord require of you but to act justly, love mercy and to walk humbly with your God." The audience for the challenge can be viewed at multiple levels, from the individual believer to the global church.

[17] Author observation, Lawrence Temfwe visit to Calvin College, Grand Rapids, Michigan, October 17, 2007.

[18] One example is Calvary Church in Grand Rapids, Michigan. For more information see http://www.calvarygr.com/ministries/missions.

[19] Prime partners are those nongovernmental organizations, government ministries, or faith-based organizations that directly receive PEPFAR grants. These prime partners often provide smaller grants to their own local partners.

6
AIDS, Churches, and Africa's Future

AIDS presents a huge challenge to Africa, a continent where Christianity continues to gain adherents and where Christian majority countries have some of the highest HIV prevalence rates. This work has painted a complicated picture of church efforts to fight the disease. It has moved beyond negative portrayals of churches as obstructionist, moralizing, or opportunistic, while also disputing the positive view that churches are tireless do-gooders motivated by other-worldly goals. As unique civil society organizations, African churches have been incorporated into the dynamic and fluid relations of power that surround AIDS politics both at the domestic and international levels. Churches both influence and are influenced by the ambiguous politics that characterizes AIDS activities, making it hard to define them as strong or weak actors and their activities as positive or negative.

This concluding chapter has two objectives. First, I take lessons from the previous chapters to highlight the ambiguous role of churches in AIDS efforts. In doing so, I suggest paths of future research for scholars interested in churches, AIDS, and Africa. I also propose questions for donors, international nongovernmental organizations, and Western congregations in their interactions with African churches. The second part of the chapter asks what the ambiguous role of churches in AIDS politics means for the churches themselves. How might churches take the lessons learned from AIDS programs and apply them to other challenges the continent faces?

Lessons in Ambiguity

When I assert that churches' role in AIDS politics is ambiguous, I do not mean we know nothing about their activities. Rather, the concept of ambiguity highlights the dynamic nature of church actions, the complicated factors that both strengthen and weaken church AIDS mobilization, and the disunity that is displayed at times among churches over proposed AIDS responses. Churches are caught in a complex political web, making clarity in their role and simplicity in analysis difficult.[1] As Chapter 2 demonstrated, churches range in their AIDS activities from those that have done nothing to those that tackled the disease soon after it appeared in Africa, with responses potentially including care, support, treatment, prevention, advocacy, and/or stigma reduction activities (see Table 2.1). Chapters 3, 4, and 5 then analyzed the variables that shaped those responses.

Chapter 3 highlighted the role of resources in AIDS activities, focusing on the ways non-monetary variables such as biblical frameworks, church hierarchies, coalitions, and pastoral leadership can mobilize or hinder AIDS activities. Through its analysis, Chapter 3 highlights some reasons why the churches' role on AIDS has been ambiguous. Churches lack a common biblical frame for mobilizing against AIDS, a fact that limits identity formation and hampers unified actions. While potentially beneficial, inter-religious coalitions rooted in equal partnerships and church cooperation with people living with HIV/AIDS have been minimal. And while the relative autonomy of Pentecostal pastors in decision making can help them to mobilize church members, build ties to donors, and forge relationships with congregations in industrialized countries, this autonomy can also threaten AIDS mobilization. With few checks on their power, some of these church leaders may compete with other pastors for resources, develop cozy relations with the state, or combatively challenge the AIDS regime.

Chapter 4 asserts that churches are engaged in forms of political activism on AIDS, even if they deny they are "playing politics." Unlike Western activism with its protests, direct lobbying, or campaigning for candidates, African church AIDS activism utilizes symbolic statements by high-level church officials, behind-the-scenes conversations between local officials and pastors, or church representation on national AIDS policy-making boards to influence state policies. As with any social movement, church mobilization on AIDS capitalizes on past political experiences: many churches that engaged in the pro-democracy movements of the 1990s mobilized on AIDS. On the other hand, it is unclear that a country's broad political environment facilitates or hampers church AIDS activities.

Ambiguity also characterizes the ways that African churches and the state interact on AIDS. In some ways, African churches appear to have the "upper hand" in this relationship: they possess power because they are believed to be able to mediate between the visible, physical realm and the unseen, but powerful spiritual realm (Ellis and ter Haar 1998).

This spiritual role heightens their leaders' moral authority and makes it difficult for church opponents to openly criticize the churches. Furthermore, Catholic and mainline Protestant churches have historic, in-depth experiences with health care provision, and donor funding may further increase the autonomy and capacity of churches. Churches seem powerful compared with the African state, which often has limited capacity, lacks legitimacy with citizens, and exhibits pervasive neopatrimonalism and corruption (van de Walle 2001).

Yet, the state remains a powerful force in AIDS politics. As Chapter 4 showed, it receives a large share of Global Fund grants, and it has the legal command to pass policies to address AIDS. The state also can offer positions of patronage on national AIDS councils or CCMs to forge ties to civil society organizations (van de Walle 2001; Englebert 2009). These factors may make the vast majority of churches hesitant to publicly push the state to combat poverty, economic inequality, and corruption, all structural variables that hamper the AIDS fight.[2] Several interviews demonstrated the ambiguity in church-state relations. For example, after bemoaning how the state had set condom policy without church input, one respondent then praised church-state cooperation on the Ghana AIDS Commission (Interview 47). To further complicate the picture, church-state interactions on AIDS vary across time and place. Some Ugandan religious leaders said that the state did not actively engage religious leaders in policy-making (IRCU 2010), while Zambian informants reported the opposite (Interviews 7, 13, 15). Yet another Zambian reported that in the past the state did not work with the church on AIDS, but now does (Interview 25).

Chapter 5 situates church AIDS actions in the context of increased global interest in AIDS during the new millennium. The chapter portrays churches as both weak and strong players in their interactions with donors. As the Compassion Campaign illustrated, church AIDS activities may rise and fall with donor priorities. On the other hand, churches might use donor funding to gain greater autonomy and build capacity, a pattern more evident with CHAZ. As the Makerere Community Church illustrates, donor-church relations are dynamic and complicated. The church received Global Fund money, but its pastor criticizes the AIDS regime. Its pastor testified in a US congressional committee in 2005, but in 2010 he was implicitly criticized when the US president urged Uganda to not pass its proposed anti-homosexual legislation.

Chapter 5 also makes problematic the assertion that churches developed AIDS programs solely to access donor money. While no one doubts that the "flood of donations" and the "lure of AIDS money" have created the conditions for the establishment of nongovernmental organizations working on AIDS (*Observer*, October 25, 2009), the picture is more complicated. Chapter 5 showed that donor money does matter for church AIDS activities, and it has the potential to affect church accountability, dependence, and program sustainability. However, global ideals, African church participation in ecumenical organizations and cross-national networks, and personal relationships between African and Western churches further condition AIDS activities. For example, when global church leaders such as Pope John Paul II and Kwesi Dickson of the All Africa Conference of Churches spoke openly about the disease, they gave local and national church leaders the "political cover" and religious legitimacy to address AIDS (Interviews 2, 25, 35, 49).

What future paths of scholarly inquiry emerge from these lessons? What cautionary notes might practitioners draw from this study? Future scholarship needs to further analyze the ways that relationships between churches and donors influence the internal decision making and leadership accountability within churches. Some studies of civil society organizations have shown that donor connections negatively affect participation and accountability in groups (Patterson 1998; Fatton 1995). Yet, do some aspects of churches (such as their mission-orientation or an emphasis on the equality of believers) prevent such corruption? On the other hand, does the high respect that church members give pastors mean that donor funding presents new opportunities for corruption?

A broader line of inquiry relates to the ways that African churches have (or have not) been incorporated into a global social movement against AIDS. Studies of the global AIDS movement have paid limited attention to religious actors and particularly those actors in Africa (Smith and Siplon 2006; Behrman 2004). The social movement paradigm, and particularly its recent incorporation into African studies (Ellis and van Kessel 2009), provides opportunities to question how actors frame AIDS in order to mobilize both religious and secular activists. Since identity creation is crucial in social movements, what symbols or words might create a broader sense of unity against the pandemic? Greater analysis of inter-religious or religious-secular cooperation to fight AIDS would inform such questions.

This book also provides lessons for practitioners. First, it demonstrates that church leadership is a crucial factor in AIDS efforts; pastors may urge or hamper church responses through public or private actions. Both secular and faith-based donors must find creative ways to support pastoral leadership while also holding these leaders accountable. Pastors need continuous information about HIV transmission, stigma reduction, and ARV treatment programs in order to remain vested in the issue. Ghana's Compassion Campaign showed that without the continued engagement of pastors, their leadership on AIDS declined and citizens' concern about AIDS waned (Interviews 29, 36, 47). Recognizing the central role of church leaders does not mean, however, that practitioners must always agree with pastors' positions or work with church leaders whose rhetoric and actions make compromise difficult. While seeking common ground is ideal, there may be times when tensions between pastors who challenge major components of the AIDS regime and secular AIDS activists, donor officials, and people living with HIV/AIDS make collaboration difficult.

Second, donors, international nongovernmental organizations, and Western churches that work with African churches need to pay attention to structures of church governance. The Catholic Church's well-established and well-resourced secretariats facilitated early and broad AIDS efforts. On the other hand, church autonomy and centralization of power around the pastor, a pattern in many New Independent churches, may allow pastors to be entrepreneurial but it also may limit their accountability. External partners must appreciate how the internal rules and structures of organizations affect those groups' ability to effectively and legitimately shape outcomes.

A third lesson is that international secular and religious organizations that seek to work with African churches must not approach these partnerships uncritically. Even though churches use moral rhetoric, they remain social organizations shaped by power dynamics. Some of the literature on faith-based organizations has shied away from analysis of power and political decision-making processes, but external partners must be willing to question how these dynamics affect access to resources and representation within churches (Marshall and van Saanen 2007). Ties to external donors may exacerbate these issues, if competition over funding leads to jealousy or rivalries (Uvin 1998). In Zambia, for example, some church AIDS workers assert that while material resources have benefited CHAZ, they have not always trickled down to congregations to support pastoral training or capacity building (Interviews 1, 9, 16). On the other hand, because it needs to demonstrate accountability to its external partners, CHAZ may not give some local churches funding because they lack capacity (FBO Roundtable 2009). The external partners of African churches must be cognizant of such dynamics.

External partners also must urge strong inner-church institutions to encourage accountability, and they must help churches to develop these institutions. As they work to foster transparency and accountability, external actors must be willing to investigate their *own* patterns of communication and decision making with African churches. While there have been some analyses of transparency and accountability within donor programs such as PEPFAR, there is little research on the ways international nongovernmental organizations and Western congregations interact with African churches (Bruckner 2010). Julie Hearn (2002) reports that accountability within the new, ad hoc relationships between American evangelical churches and individual African churches has been limited, but scholars and practitioners need more details about how power dynamics influence these relationships. Such insights could help increase program effectiveness and prevent Western partners from approaching AIDS with the sometimes patronizing, short-term goal of "fixing the problem" (Interviews 55, 56).

In summary, churches are situated within a complicated web of dynamic processes that influence their AIDS activities. Their complex and diverse interactions with other religious leaders, people living with HIV/AIDS, and state officials shape the churches' desire and ability to combat AIDS. Their lack of coherent biblical frame for understanding AIDS and mobilizing action contributes to a variety of AIDS activities among churches. The central role of pastoral leadership presents opportunities for entrepreneurship on AIDS, but may also limit pastors' accountability. And churches, while seeking access to donor money, may also be driven to address AIDS by historic ties to ecumenical organizations, personal networks, and the desire for independency in global Christianity.

A New Role or More of the Same?

AIDS is not the only problem Africa faces: poverty, gender inequality, corruption, infectious diseases, war, crime, and unemployment are only a few of the others. Have churches transferred the lessons from their experiences with AIDS to other issues? I first suggest the ways that AIDS involvement has influenced churches. I then examine church efforts to address some of the continent's other problems. The final analysis reveals that the current and future role of Africa's churches in the continent's development is complicated and uncertain.

The Meaning of the AIDS Fight for Africa's Churches

Church AIDS efforts have had three broad effects on African churches. First, the inability or unwillingness of some African churches to address the disease has negatively affected the legitimacy of *all* church AIDS efforts. AIDS activists, scholars, and secular AIDS organizations have criticized African churches for ignoring the disease or for responding too slowly to the crisis (Epstein 2007; Csete 2007). Even the churches' own AIDS organizers have echoed these critiques (Interviews 1, 2, 9, 14, 16, 26, 35, 36, 47, 50). Additionally, African churches have been viewed with suspicion, because some have challenged the AIDS regime. While many churches do not like aspects of the regime (such as condom distribution), most recognize the need for various approaches to HIV prevention (Uganda Religious Leaders 2010; Interview 7). The minority of pastors who have used combative language and actions against the regime may have hampered opportunities for collaboration. To facilitate better cooperation and communication between churches on the one hand, and donors, secular AIDS groups, and AIDS experts on the other, African churches must be willing to hold their brethren accountable if they stigmatize people living with HIV/AIDS, criticize established scientific findings, or deny the existence of AIDS in the church. There is some evidence that African churches (particularly national ecumenical councils) have begun to distance themselves from churches and pastors engaging in such negative actions (*Public Agenda*, December 10, 2007; *Arusha Times*, August 18, 2007; *New Vision,* August 29, 2007).

Second, according to some interviewees, African church efforts on AIDS have begun to empower some church members and institutions.[3] One Zambian discussed how church members have become more willing to ask local government officials about resources for water and health care because of the confidence they had gained through AIDS work (Interview 24). An official with a global ecumenical organization asserted that through congregational discussions of members' health challenges, such as the lack of available ARVs at local clinics, churchgoers have realized the need to meet with local government officials. Through this lobbying, church members have gained a greater sense of citizen rights and responsibilities (Interview 61). Similarly, some home-based care volunteers report greater respect in the community because of their AIDS expertise. One Mozambican worker said, "When someone is sick, the community leaders come to us for help. Before we were nobodies. So now we feel good; we feel honoured" (quoted in Iliffe 2006, 107; see also Vander Meulen 2010). A volunteer child advocate with the Kamwokya Christian Caring Community echoed this sentiment when he said the reason he does his work is because it gives him recognition, respect, and new friends in his community.[4]

Participation in "seemingly apolitical matters" such as AIDS programs may develop individuals' skills in organizing, budgeting, strategic planning, coordinating volunteers, and public speaking (VonDoepp 1998; see also Verba, Schlozman, and Brady 1995). And church members may grow in their exposure to and knowledge about complex societal problems. Knowledge has led some parishioners to realize they cannot focus solely on spiritual issues when physical suffering is everywhere (Interview 41). The following anecdote from the Northmead Assembly of God Church illustrates this rise in social consciousness.

In the late 1990s, several sex workers had begun to conduct business near the Northmead church. To avoid exposing church members to the women and their clients, church officers cancelled evening worship services. However, after a youth pastor found a woman and her client engaging in sexual relations outside the church door early one morning, congregants decided they could no longer ignore the issue and they began an outreach program. While members first approached the sex workers with an attitude of condemnation, parishioners (who were mostly middle class) soon discovered how financially desperate the women were and that their ages varied greatly, with the youngest being thirteen. Members had assumed the sex workers were single, "loose" women, but several of them were married. Parishioners quickly recognized that merely preaching morality would not address the problem, so they started a six-month program to teach the women new skills and to help them establish small businesses. Not only did the program lead to a decline in the number of sex workers in the neighborhood, but it also increased congregants' awareness of community problems and their understanding of the people who face those problems. By addressing (not avoiding) the prostitution issue, members learned about complex social issues and discovered how churches can meet both spiritual and physical needs (Interview 7; Northmead Assembly of God 2009).

Churches as institutions also have been empowered, through greater access to resources and more political clout. Some informants enthusiastically described new church AIDS programs. And while some church leaders felt they had to follow donors' wishes, others thought their relations with external partners were increasingly built on mutual respect (Interviews 7, 8, 11, 24, 26, 29, 35, 36). Church recipients of donor funds have had to develop organizational capacity. Some international donors and faith-based organizations have partnered with African churches to teach their leaders report writing, basic accounting practices, and management skills. Many external partners require local churches to complete "compliance training" before they receive small grants (Interview 11). The churches also have recognized that to be eligible for money from the Global Fund, national AIDS councils, and PEPFAR's primary partners (who tend to be American nongovernmental organizations), they must develop structures for monitoring and evaluation. Church officials recognize that this has been one of the benefits of their AIDS activities and that this new-found capacity has the potential to positively influence Africa's future development (Uganda Religious Leaders 2010).

On the other hand, institutional empowerment may lead churches increasingly to resemble other civil society organizations that seek funding, power, and relevance in African society (Joshua 2009; Christiansen 2009). In their professionalization, churches may lose what some find to be their unique qualities, such as their highly motivated volunteers, spiritual mission, and holistic approaches to development. As one informant mused (Interview 61), once churches become increasingly institutionalized, will they be willing to give up material resources and power, if they recognize how these assets may undermine their spiritual mission?

The issue of remuneration for home-based care workers illustrates this perceived danger. Donors and international nongovernmental organizations are increasingly providing local faith-based and community-based organizations money to pay home-based care workers. Supporters of these payments assert that because home-based care workers spend on average three hours per day on care, they should be compensated for lost income-earning opportunities (Interviews 10, 11, 12; Iliffe 2006, 101-106). Yet, for some religious and secular actors, such remuneration seems to contradict the belief that church members are willing to give time and energy to the sick, hungry, poor, and marginalized (Marshall and van Saanen 2007; Vander Meulen 2010). Does remuneration for home-based care workers make churches just like any other nongovernmental organization? If only some home-based care programs pay workers will the jealousy that emerges divide the Christian community? (Interview 10) How churches ultimately resolve these issues may define how they integrate their religious perspectives on health, development, and Christian service with their engagement in a society characterized by high poverty and limited economic opportunities.

Third, AIDS work has led some churches to become more involved in politics. As Chapter 4 demonstrated, Catholic and mainline Protestants were the predominant church actors in the pro-democracy movements of the 1990s. Since then, some established and new Pentecostal churches have joined the Old Mission churches in playing a political role. As Pentecostal churches have developed community outreach programs on AIDS, education, and poverty reduction, they have recognized the need for funding, policy changes, and church representation in policy-making (Miller and Yamamori 2007). They also have gained greater exposure to the ways corruption, nepotism, and patronage affect their ability to meet their objectives. While these newer churches' political involvement may have allowed some church leaders to participate in these nefarious practices, it has led others to publicly speak against them (Ranger 2008).

My point is not to make a normative judgment on the positive or negative implications of church political participation. Rather, I make an empirical observation: African churches are more involved in politics than in the past, and the New Mission and New Independent churches have become more incorporated into policy-making. While some of these churches (particularly the Pentecostals) might deny that they are "playing politics," their efforts to influence state and donor funding decisions and AIDS policies (particularly HIV prevention programs) engage deeply *political* questions about power, representation, and societal values. But this new role is not clearly defined. Few African churches have developed a framework for political involvement that will urge believers to participate in political activities that foster social justice; instead, participation is often understood in terms of narrow self-interest (Carpenter 2009).

Few churches also have questioned how their political participation and growing institutional capacity may affect their relations with the African state or may shape the nature of the state itself. The capacity and voice of churches may increasingly put them at odds with the state. On the positive side, strong, autonomous civil society organizations like churches may challenge the state to become more accountable and effective. On the other hand, these non-state actors may draw resources (such as donor funds), personnel, and legitimacy away from the state, further weakening it. As one informant pointed out, this latter scenario is problematic because Africa's long-term development requires an accountable, transparent state with the ability to address the continent's problems of poverty, disease, unemployment, and economic inequality. African nongovernmental organizations and their international partners cannot meet these demands in a comprehensive manner (Interview 61). The dialectic relationship between churches and the state will shape Africa's long-term development.

Churches and the Continent's Future Development

Despite their AIDS activities, it is uncertain that the majority of churches in either Africa or the West have applied lessons from their AIDS work to fight other social inequalities and global injustices that make AIDS so devastating for Africa. While cross-national efforts such as the Micah Challenge or the Ecumenical Advocacy Alliance have sought to raise awareness about global inequities in trade and development spending, they have given less attention to other problems such as the West's recruitment of African health care workers and the huge inefficiencies in US foreign aid programs (Mills et al. 2008; Riddell 2008). Mobilizing and educating members of Western churches to address the structural obstacles that negatively affect the continent presents political and theological challenges (Interviews 54, 55, 56).

Similarly, one interview criticized African churches for their inability or unwillingness to act as a prophetic voice against underdevelopment and inequality:

> I mean speaking out for more than just AIDS, the one issue, but for the things that make people vulnerable to AIDS, like issues of fair trade, poverty, [and] gender inequality. I like to quote Pasteur, 'The virus is nothing; the terrain is everything.' And the church needs to focus more on the terrain. (Interview 23)

To illustrate the limited way African churches have applied their organizational and political skills from their AIDS work to the continent's other problems, I examine church mobilization on gender-based violence, violence against children, and morbidity and mortality caused by malaria and diarrhea. I focus on these problems for three reasons. First, these issues lack simple technical answers; solving them requires that well-respected and well-organized institutions such as churches promote education and urge changes in individual behavior. Second, biblical interpretations by church leaders shape congregants' views on gender norms, family roles, and compassion for the sick, all themes clearly related to the issues of violence and disease. Third, these problems are closely linked to AIDS. Gender inequality can make women more economically dependent on men, more likely to have multiple sexual partners, and more likely to stay in abusive relationships, all factors that increase women's vulnerability to HIV infection. Child sexual abuse increases the risk of HIV transmission for victims (Oppong, Oppong, and Odotei 2006; Epstein 2007; Nabalonzi

2000; CIDA n.d.). HIV-positive pregnant women with malaria face serious complications in pregnancy, and malaria and water-borne diseases make individuals more vulnerable to HIV infection (Stillwaggon 2006).

First, few African churches have challenged the larger societal attitudes and practices that demean and dehumanize women and put them at risk for HIV infection, injury, and death (Kelly 2007, 15). African theologians such as Ezra Chitando (2007), Barbara Schmid (2006), Beverley Haddad (2002, 2005), and members of the Circle of Concerned African Women Theologians (2002) have repeatedly raised this limitation in their analyses of church AIDS activities. By ignoring or denying the issue, the majority of African church leaders seem out of touch with the realities of society. For example, in Zambia, more than 50 percent of women reported being beaten and physically mistreated since the age of fifteen, and 24 percent reported physical violence in the last year. Eighty-five percent of women believed that it is justifiable for a husband to beat his wife if she neglects a child or argues with him (Zambian Government 2002). Since Zambia is 82 percent Christian, one can assume that this high level of gender-based violence affects churchgoers and congregational life. Yet, according to several interviewees, denial in churches is prevalent (Interviews 1, 2, 11, 23). One informant complained: "Some churches refuse to make domestic violence—physical and emotional—an issue. This is true even though the church is predominantly made up of women" (Interview 12).

Churches also have been noticeably silent on what Paul Farmer (2005) terms the "structural violence" found in Africa's inadequate health care systems, an injustice which disproportionately affects pregnant women and allows 250,000 of them to die annually from complications in pregnancy and childbirth. An African woman faces a 1-in-13 chance of dying in childbirth, compared to a 1-in-4,100 chance for a woman in an industrialized country. Many of these deaths could be prevented by providing access to skilled care at delivery, encouraging girls to stay in school (to prevent early pregnancy), and enforcing minimal legal ages for marriage (again, to prevent early pregnancy) (UNICEF 2009b). While churches face resource and logistical challenges in building health care infrastructure or training birth attendants, they can use their moral authority to publicly call attention to maternal mortality and to support later marriage for girls. Since marriage and family are often framed in light of biblical messages, church leaders are uniquely placed to educate parishioners on the dangers of girls' early marriage.

There seems to be a divide between those African theologians and ecumenical organizations that have begun to address these gender-related inequalities and church leaders at the national and local levels who have remained relatively silent on these issues. The EHAIA program of the World Council of Churches condemns the patterns of male sexual behavior that may put women at risk for HIV infection (Chitando 2007). The World Council of Churches has called for greater advocacy on maternal morality and unequal access to health services for women and children (World Council of Churches 2005a). Yet, the number of local pastors who will speak openly on these issues from the pulpit remains small (Interviews 1, 2, 16, 20, 35, 43, 50, 58). This divide leads to the perception that the entire church has no interest in these issues, and that by ignoring them, the church may even help perpetuate these problems. For example, the United Nations Special Rapporteur on Violence against Women explicitly stated in 2008 that religious institutions' support for violence against women is widespread throughout Africa (*Public Agenda*, December 5, 2008).

Few churches have applied the skills gained from their AIDS efforts to address the second problem, the physical and sexual abuse of children. While data on violence against children is sparse, experts have documented widespread physical and/or psychological aggression against Africa's children. Over 90 percent of children between two and fourteen years old in Cameroon, Sierra Leone, Togo, Côte d'Ivoire, and Ghana experience aggression (UNICEF 2010). Roughly 5 percent of African children experience child sexual abuse, with schools being one of the most common venues for these atrocities (Lalor 2004). For example, 38 percent of South Africa's young rape victims point to a teacher or principal as the perpetrator (Kielland and Tovo 2006, 136).[5]

Despite debates about cultural understandings of parenting and child discipline, no society condones child sexual abuse or violence against its weakest members. Yet, in poor countries, it is often children without adult protectors—"[those with] lowest status in the pecking order: stepchildren, orphans, [domestic] servants, and apprentices"—who experience the most egregious forms of violence (Kielland and Tovo 2006, 134).

Musa Dube (2002) asserts that biblical commands to protect the weak and marginalized must lead churches to speak for child victims of violence and sexual abuse. While some churches have worked with international faith-based organizations to combat this violence, African church leaders have been relatively silent on this topic.[6] In contrast to the thousands of news articles between 1995 and 2008 that I found in the

LexisNexis Academic database search on churches and HIV/AIDS, there were only about a dozen stories about churches and their efforts to combat violence against children. Unwillingness to get involved in family relationships, children's limited voice in African societies that are typically defined by patriarchy and gerontocracy, and biblical interpretations that give adults ultimate power over children hamper church actions (Kielland and Tovo 2006, 147).[7] Yet, as the Zimbabwean theologian and activist Ezra Chitando (2007, 33-34) writes, "African churches must play a leading role in denouncing the abuse of children, including the abuse of children within their own institutions."

Third, few African churches have applied skills from their AIDS campaigns to the prevention of malaria and diarrhea, two health problems that kill millions of Africans annually. The World Health Organization estimates that diarrhea caused 16 percent of the deaths of African children under the age of five between 2000 and 2003 (Powder 2006). Globally, in 2008, diarrhea that resulted from bacteria, parasites, and viruses was the second biggest childhood killer, leading to roughly 2.5 million deaths. In the same year, approximately 900,000 Africans died of malaria, a disease which constitutes 10 percent of Africa's overall disease burden and 40 percent of its public health expenditure. While deaths from malaria and diarrhea are often believed to be part of life in Africa, this outcome is not inevitable. With increased hand washing, exclusive breastfeeding, awareness of the dangers of open defecation, and education on fluid replacement, diarrhea deaths can decrease. Similarly, the use of insecticide-treated bed nets for children and pregnant women can cut the number of malaria deaths (UNICEF 2009a; PMI 2009; Roll Back Malaria 2009). The adoption of such behaviors requires community mobilization and education. Well-respected and highly trusted community leaders such as pastors can use faith teachings on physical and spiritual health to urge citizens to adopt these public health practices. Yet few religious leaders with experience in AIDS awareness campaigns have become publicly involved on malaria (Marshall 2008b). In fact, one Ghanaian informant laughed when I asked if church leaders ever discussed malaria prevention with parishioners in sermons or church meetings (Interview 26). In recent years, governments and donors have called for increased religious involvement in malaria prevention; in 2008, for example, the Zambian health minister symbolically used a prayer service to implore churches to tackle the disease (*Times of Zambia*, November 26, 2008).

The complex, dynamic nature of church AIDS responses, the churches' ambiguous role in the politics of AIDS, and their inability to transfer advocacy, mobilization, and organizational lessons from the

AIDS fight to other pressing issues may bring despair to Christians who yearn for a global church that promotes social justice, speaks for the weak, and cares for the powerless. One could add to this pessimism the decline in media coverage and political attention to AIDS and the increasingly loud complaint from public health officials that the pandemic has drawn needed financial resources from other pressing health concerns (*Observer*, October 25, 2009). Major scientific developments such as an AIDS vaccine seem distant, while HIV resistance to first- and second-line ARVs continues to rise in Africa (*Yahoo News*, December 30, 2009).[8] Even as HIV prevention campaigns show some positive effects, there were 1.9 million new HIV infections in Africa in 2008 (UNAIDS 2009; UNAIDS 2010b). And as Ghanaian and Zambian informants bemoaned, "People are just tired of hearing about AIDS" (Interviews 30, 36, 58).

Despite this reality and the numerous challenges looming over the African continent, in my numerous conversations with both religious and secular actors involved with AIDS in Africa, I was often struck by a lack of despondency. While they acknowledged that many factors both urged and prevented churches from acting on AIDS or led the church to half-hearted efforts, and while they saw the challenges presented by a changing global agenda and limited scientific breakthroughs, they remained optimistic. They believed that long after donor AIDS programs ended and "suitcase NGOs" shut their doors, the church would remain to fight AIDS and other social problems, however imperfectly (FBO Roundtable 2009; Interviews 2, 7, 8, 10, 11, 15, 16, 24, 25, 31, 33, 35, 37, 45, 54, 60). These respondents' views may soon be tested, since by 2010 it appeared that AIDS had declined greatly in importance on the global political agenda. In that year, funding for PEPFAR stagnated; the American commitment to the Global Fund declined by $50 million; Global Fund grants were on average 12 percent smaller than in 2009; and the World Bank MAP Initiative was scheduled to end (*New York Times*, May 9, 2010).

Given this scenario, churches will no doubt continue to play a role, however ambiguous, in AIDS politics. Whether this is a role Christians and non-Christians in Africa and the West *want* the church to play is not the question. Given the weakness of the African state, the intersection of spiritual and material life in Africa, and the continuous spread of Christianity on the continent, the churches will no doubt remain crucial societal institutions. AIDS presents African churches with "a moment of truth … and a moment of grace and opportunity" (Maluleke 2001, 130). How churches act in this historic moment will depend on their ability to appreciate their political role, to adapt to fluid international interest in the disease and in the continent, and to remain hopeful.

---

[1] I am grateful to Roland Hoksbergen for guiding my thinking on this point.

[2] The Catholic Church has been most vocal on these structural issues. The case of Catholic leaders in Zambia in Chapter 4 provides one illustration.

[3] Kenly Fenio (2009) finds some evidence of this empowerment among participants in secular AIDS groups in Mozambique.

[4] Author observations, visit to Kamwokya Christian Caring Community, Kampala, Uganda, July 7, 2010.

[5] The widespread sexual abuse scandal in the Catholic Church in the United States demonstrates that church leaders and parishioners in industrialized countries do not protect children any more than their counterparts in developing nations.

[6] For example, International Needs Network, an American organization that partners with African churches, has helped children in the Volta Region of Ghana who were former slaves to fetish priests (or *trokosi*) to gain educational and income-generating opportunities. Patience Vormawor, International Needs Network, presentation to Calvin College semester program, Accra, Ghana, November 10, 2008.

[7] Exodus 20:12 (the commandment to honor one's father and mother) and Proverbs 13:24 (the statement that sparing physical discipline—"the rod"—reflects a lack of love for one's child) are two examples of Bible verses used to support violence against children.

[8] In 2010, scientists reported that women in a South African clinical trial who used a vaginal microbicidal gel that contained the antiretroviral medication tenofovir were 39 percent less likely to contract HIV than women using a placebo. While the research was preliminary, it provided hope for future scientific breakthroughs (*New York Times*, July 19, 2010).

Interviews

1. Denominational AIDS Coordinator, Lusaka, August 6, 2007
2. Official with Global Ecumenical Organization, Lusaka, August 7, 2007
3. Zambian Professor, Lusaka, August 12, 2007
4. Donor Official, Lusaka, August 13, 2007
5. Zambian Government Official, Lusaka, August 14, 2007
6. Donor Official, Lusaka, August 14, 2007
7. Zambian Faith-Based Organization Leader, Lusaka, August 14, 2007
8. Zambian Faith-Based Organization Leader, Lusaka, August 14, 2007
9. Denominational AIDS Coordinator, Lusaka, August 14, 2007
10. Denominational AIDS Coordinator, Lusaka, August 13, 2007
11. Official with International Faith-Based Organization, Lusaka, August 15, 2007
12. Official with International Faith-Based Organization, Lusaka, August 15, 2007
13. Donor Official, Lusaka, August 15, 2007
14. Zambian Ecumenical AIDS Coordinator, Lusaka, August 15, 2007
15. Zambian Faith-Based Organization Leader, Lusaka, August 16, 2007
16. Zambian Ecumenical AIDS Coordinator, Lusaka, August 16, 2007
17. Zambian Faith-Based Organization Leader, Lusaka, August 17, 2007
18. Zambian Professor, Lusaka, August 17, 2007
19. Zambian AIDS Nongovernmental Organization Official, Lusaka, August 17, 2007
20. Zambian AIDS Nongovernmental Organization Official, Lusaka, August 20, 2007
21. Zambian AIDS Nongovernmental Organization Official, Lusaka, August 20, 2007
22. Zambian AIDS Nongovernmental Organization Official, Lusaka, August 20, 2007
23. Denominational AIDS Official, Lusaka, August 20, 2007

24. Zambian Faith-Based Organization Leader, Lusaka, October 24, 2007 (phone interview)
25. Official with Global Ecumenical Organization, Nairobi, February 15, 2008 (phone interview)
26. Former Denominational Health Coordinator, Accra, November 10, 2008
27. Ghanaian Government Official, Accra, October 10, 2008
28. Ghanaian AIDS Nongovernmental Organization Official, Accra, October 14, 2008
29. Denominational AIDS Coordinator, Accra, September 2, 2008
30. Former Denominational AIDS Coordinator, Kumasi, December 2, 2008
31. Ghanaian Pastor and AIDS Counselor, Accra, November 25, 2008
32. Ghanaian Pastor, Accra, November 18, 2008
33. Ghanaian Pastor, Accra, September 27, 2008
34. Donor Official, Accra, October 8, 2008
35. Denominational AIDS Coordinator, Accra, October 21, 2008
36. Ghanaian Faith-Based Organization Youth Worker, Accra, August 29, 2008
37. Ghanaian Pastor, Accra, November 11, 2008
38. Ghanaian Professor, Accra, October 1, 2008
39. Ghanaian AIDS Nongovernmental Organization Official, Accra, October 10, 2008
40. International Nongovernmental Organization Official, Accra, August 31, 2008
41. Denominational AIDS Coordinator, Accra, September 25, 2008
42. Ghanaian Pastor, Accra, October 14, 2008
43. Former Ghanaian Nongovernmental Organization Official, Accra, November 30, 2008
44. Official with Global Ecumenical Organization, Accra, December 18, 2008 (written correspondence)
45. Denominational Health Coordinator, Accra, September 25, 2008
46. Denominational Women's Coordinator, Accra, December 4, 2008
47. Ghanaian Pastor, Accra, August 27, 2008
48. AIDS Nongovernmental Organization Official, Accra, November 18, 2008
49. Former Denominational Representative, Accra, August 29, 2008
50. Former Denominational AIDS Coordinator, Accra, September 24, 2008
51. Ghanaian Faith-Based Organization Official, Kumasi, December 2, 2008

52. International Nongovernmental Organization Official, Accra, October 5, 2008
53. Official with Global Ecumenical Organization, Grand Rapids, MI, May 21, 2008
54. International Faith-Based Organization Official, Washington, DC, March 18, 2005
55. International Faith-Based Organization Official, Grand Rapids, MI, February 13, 2008
56. International Faith-Based Organization Official, San Francisco, CA, March 28, 2008
57. Former Bilateral Donor Official, Washington, DC, April 15, 2005
58. Denominational AIDS coordinator, Lusaka, April 13, 2009
59. International AIDS researcher, Lusaka, April 13, 2009
60. Zambian physician, Lusaka, April 14, 2009
61. Official with African Ecumenical Organization, Grand Rapids, MI, June 24, 2010
62. Official with Ugandan Faith-Based Organization, Kampala, July 8, 2010

Acronyms

ACT UP	AIDS Coalition to Unleash Power
ADRA	Adventist Development and Relief Agency
AIDS	Acquired Immunodeficiency Syndrome
ANERELA+	African Network of Religious Leaders Living with or Affected by HIV and AIDS
ARV	Antiretroviral
CCM	Country Coordinating Mechanism
CHAG	Christian Health Association of Ghana
CHAZ	Churches Health Association of Zambia
CIDA	Canadian International Development Agency
DGAAN	DuPage Glocal AIDS Action Network
EHAIA	Ecumenical HIV and AIDS Initiative in Africa
FBO	Faith-Based Organization
GIPA	Greater Involvement of People Living with HIV/AIDS
Health GAP	Health Global Access Project
HIV	Human Immunodeficiency Virus
MAP	Multi-Country AIDS Program (World Bank)
NAC	National HIV/AIDS/STI/TB Council (Zambia)
NETACT	Network for African Congregational Theology
NGO	Nongovernmental Organization
PEPFAR	President's Emergency Plan for AIDS Relief (United States)
PMI	President's Malaria Initiative (United States)
TB	Tuberculosis
UN	United Nations
UNAIDS	Joint United Nations Program on HIV/AIDS
UNDP	United Nations Development Program
USAID	United States Agency for International Development
UNICEF	The United Nations Children's Fund
WARC	World Alliance of Reformed Churches
WCC	World Council of Churches

WEA	World Evangelical Alliance
WHO	World Health Organization
ZINGO	Zambia Interfaith Networking Group on HIV/AIDS

Bibliography

AACC. *See* All Africa Conference of Churches.

ACHA. *See* Africa Christian Health Association.

Adamczyk, Amy. 2010. Religion and Health-Related Social Activism in Sub-Saharan Africa. Paper Presented at the AIDS, Religion and Social Activism Workshop, International Research Network on AIDS and Religion in Africa, Makerere University, Kampala, July 8.

Addai, Isaac. 2000. Religious Affiliation and Sexual Initiation among Ghanaian Women. *Review of Religious Research* 41 (3): 328-343.

Africa Christian Health Association. 2009. Report of the Fourth Biennial Conference. Kampala, 22-27 February. http://www.africachap.org/x5/images/stories/2009%20%20conference%20report%20-final1.pdf.

African Network of Religious Leaders Living with or Affected by HIV and AIDS. 2006. *General Report*. Nairobi: ANERELA+.

African Religious Health Assets Program. 2006. *Appreciating Assets: The Contribution of Religion to Universal Access in Africa*. Report for the World Health Organization. Cape Town: ARHAP.

Afrobarometer. 2004. *Public Opinion and HIV/AIDS: Facing Up to the Future?* Briefing Paper 12. http://www.afrobarometer.org/papers/AfrobriefNo12.pdf.

------. 2005. *Round 3 Afrobarometer Survey in Zambia*. Summary of Results. http://www.afrobarometer.org/Summary%20of%20Results/Round%203/zam-R3SOR-23jan07-final.pdf.

------. 2009. *Are Democratic Citizens Emerging in Africa?* Executive Survey. Briefing Paper 70. http://www.afrobarometer.org/papers/AfrobriefNo70_21may09.pdf.

Agadjanian, Victor, and Soma Sen. 2007. Promises and Challenges of Faith-Based AIDS Care and Support in Mozambique. *American Journal of Public Health* 97 (2): 362-366.

Akanji, Olajide. 2009. Faith-Based Organizations and HIV/AIDS Advocacy in Nigeria: The Case of the Redeemed Christian Church of God. Paper presented to the Conference of the International Research Network on Religion and AIDS in Africa, Lusaka, Zambia, April 15-17.

All Africa Conference of Churches. 2008. About Us. http://www.aacc-ceta.org/en/default2.asp?active_page_id=57.

Allen, Susan, Etienne Karita, Elwyn Chomba, David Roth, Joseph Telfair, Isaac Zulu, Leslie Clark, Nzali Kancheya, Martha Conkling, Rob Stephenson, Brigitte Bekan, Katherine Kimbrell, Steven Dunham, Faith Henderson, Moses Sinkala, Michel Carael, and Alan Haworth. 2007. Promotion of

Couples' Voluntary Counseling and Testing for HIV Through Influential Networks in Two African Capital Cities. *BMC Public Health* 7 (349): 1-10.

Alsan, Marcella. 2006. Catholic Church Condom Prohibition Comes Face to Face with Reality of AIDS in Africa. *Commonweal Magazine: A Review of Religion, Politics, and Culture.* http://www.catholic.org/international/international_story.php?id=19561.

ANERELA+. *See* African Network of Religious Leaders Living with or Affected by HIV and AIDS.

Apostolic Faith Church. 2009. About Us. http://www.apostolicfaith.org/aboutus.

ARHAP. *See* African Religious Health Assets Program.

Asamoah-Gyadu, J. Kwabena. 2005a. "Christ is the Answer": What Is the Question? A Ghana Airways Prayer Vigil and Its Implications for Religion, Evil and Public Space. *Journal of Religion in Africa* 35 (1): 93-117.

------. 2005b. Rethinking African Worldviews of Mystical Causality: Mission and Ecclesiology in the Era of HIV/AIDS. Paper presented at the World Council of Churches/Trinity Theological Seminary Consultation on Mainstreaming HIV/AIDS in Theological Education, Trinity Theological Seminary, Legon, Ghana, June 12-18.

AVERT. 2008. Background on AIDS Orphans. http://www.avert.org/aidsorphans.htm.

------. 2009. AIDS Treatment Target and Results. http://www.avert.org/aidstarget.htm.

Azarya, Victor. 1988. Reordering State-Society Relations: Incorporation and Disengagement. In *The Precarious Balance: State and Society in Africa*, ed. Donald Rothchild and Naomi Chazan, 3-21. Boulder, CO: Westview Press.

Banda, D. T. 2007. Zambia. Presentation to the Conference of the Network for African Congregational Theology, Lusaka, Zambia, August 4-11.

Banda, Kunyima. 2009. Religion and Universal Access to Care. Presentation to the Conference of the International Research Network on Religion and AIDS in Africa, Lusaka, Zambia, April 15- 17.

Barnett, Tony, and Alan Whiteside. 2002. *AIDS in the Twenty-First Century: Disease and Globalisation.* New York: Palgrave MacMillan.

Barrett, David, and Todd Johnson. 2001a. Annual Statistical Table on Global Mission: 2001. *International Bulletin of Missionary Research* 25 (1): 24-25.

------. 2001b. *World Christian Trends AD 30 to AD 2200.* Pasadena, CA: William Careley Library.

------. 2004. Annual Statistical Table on Global Mission: 2004. *International Bulletin of Missionary Research* 28 (1): 24-25.

Barrett, David, George Kurian, and Todd Johnson. 2001. *World Christian Encyclopedia: A Comparative Survey of Churches and Religions in the Modern World.* New York: Oxford University Press.

Bates, Robert. 2008. *When Things Fell Apart: State Failure in Late-Century Africa.* New York: Cambridge University Press.

Bayart, Jean-François. 1993. *The State in Africa: The Politics of the Belly.* London: Longman.

Becker, Felicitas. 2007. The Virus and the Scriptures: Muslims and AIDS in Tanzania. *Journal of Religion in Africa* 37 (1): 16-40.

Becker, Felicitas, and P. Wenzel Geissler. 2007. Searching for Pathways in a Landscape of Death: Religion and AIDS in East Africa. *Journal of Religion in Africa* 37 (1): 1-15.

Beckley, Robert, and Jerome Koch. 2002. *The Continuing Challenge of AIDS: Clergy Responses to Patients, Friends, and Families*. Westport, CT: Auburn House.

Behrman, Greg. 2004. *The Invisible People: How the U.S. Has Slept Through the Global AIDS Pandemic, the Greatest Humanitarian Catastrophe of Our Time*. New York: Free Press.

Berg, Allison, director. 2005. *Witches in Exile*. Documentary. California Newsreel Distributor.

Berger, Peter, ed. 1999. *The Desecularization of the World: Resurgent Religion in World Politics*. Grand Rapids, MI: Eerdmans.

Black, Amy, Douglas Koopman, and Dave Ryden. 2004. *Of Little Faith: The Politics of George W. Bush's Faith-Based Initiatives*. Washington, DC: Georgetown University Press.

Blumenthal, Max. 2009. Rick Warren's Africa Problem. *The Daily Beast*. http://www.thedailybeast.com/blogs-and-stories/2009-01-07/the-truth-about-rick-warren-in-africa.

Bodewes, Christine. 2009. Perspectives on the Slums of Nairobi, Kenya: What is the Role of the Churches? Presentation to the Paul Henry Institute, Calvin College, Grand Rapids, MI, October 20.

Bongmba, Elias. 2007. *Facing a Pandemic: The African Church and the Crisis of AIDS*. Waco, TX: Baylor University Press.

Borer, Tristan. 1998. *Challenging the State: Churches as Political Actors in South Africa*. Notre Dame, IN: Notre Dame Press.

Bornstein, Erica. 2005. *The Spirit of Development: Protestant NGOs, Morality, and Economics in Zimbabwe*. Stanford, CA: Stanford University Press.

Botha, Johan. 2007. Public Witness and Public Theology. Presentation to the Conference of the Network for African Congregational Theology, Lusaka, Zambia, August 4-11.

Boulay, Marc, Ian Tweedie, and Emmanuel Fiagbey. 2008. The Effectiveness of a National Communication Campaign Using Religious Leaders to Reduce HIV-Related Stigma in Ghana. *African Journal of AIDS Research* 7 (1): 133-141.

Brain, Joy. 1997. Moving from the Margins to the Mainstream: The Roman Catholic Church. In *Christianity in South Africa: A Political, Social and Cultural History*, ed. Richard Elphick and T. R. H. Davenport, 195-210. Berkeley: University of California Press.

Bratton, Michael. 1989. Beyond the State: Civil Society and Associational Life in Africa. *World Politics* 41 (3): 407-429.

Bratton, Michael, and Wonbin Cho. 2006. *Where is Africa Going? Views from Below*. Working Paper 60. http://www.afrobarometer.org/papers/AfropaperNo60-trends.pdf.

Bratton, Michael, and Nicolas van de Walle. 1997. *Democratic Experiments in Africa*. New York: Cambridge University Press.

Bruckner, Till. 2010. The Accidental NGO and USAID Transparency Test. Article posted on Aid Watch Blog. August 18. http://aidwatchers.com/2010/08/the-accidental-ngo-and-usaid-transparency-test.

Burchardt, Marian. 2010. Interpretative Flexibility: Framing Politics, Patronage and the Limits of Autonomy in Faith-Based AIDS Activism in South Africa. Paper Presented at the AIDS, Religion and Social Activism Workshop, International Research Network on AIDS and Religion in Africa, Makerere University, Kampala, July 5.

Byamugisha, Canon Gideon. 2010. Understanding Religious Involvement in the Ugandan AIDS Response. Panel Discussion at the AIDS, Religion and Social Activism Workshop, International Research Network on AIDS and Religion in Africa, Makerere University, Kampala, July 7.

Campbell, Catherine. 2003. *"Letting Them Die": Why HIV/AIDS Prevention Programmes Fail*. Bloomington: Indiana University Press.

Canadian International Development Agency. n.d. *Socio-Economic Factors Contributing to Girl Child Abuse in Botswana*. Report for CIDA. http://www.crin.org/resources/publications/Botswana_CIDA.doc.

Carmody, Brendan. 2003. Religious Heritage and Premarital Sex in Zambia. *Journal of Theology for Southern Africa* 115 (March): 79-90.

Carpenter, Joel. 2009. Now What? Revivalist Christianity and Global South Politics. *Books & Culture* (March-April): 26-28.

Catholic Secretariat. n.d. Activities at Buduburam Refugee Settlement, Ghana. Unpublished Report. Accra, Ghana: Catholic Secretariat.

Center for Global Health Policy. 2010a. Physicians, Other Public Health Experts Decry Anti-Gay Bill in Uganda. http://sciencespeaks.wordpress.com/2010/01/19/physicians-other-public-health-experts-decry-anti-gay-bill-in-uganda.

-----. 2010b. Uganda Bill Gets a Hearing in U.S. Congress. http://sciencespeaks.wordpress.com/2010/01/22/uganda-bill-gets-a-hearing-in-u-s-congress.

Chabal, Patrick, and Jean-Pascal Daloz. 1999. *Africa Works: Disorder as Political Instrument*. Bloomington: Indiana University Press.

CHAG. *See* Christian Health Association of Ghana.

CHAZ. *See* Churches Health Association of Zambia.

Chitando, Ezra. 2007. *Acting in Hope: African Churches and HIV/AIDS*. Geneva: World Council of Churches.

Christian Council of Ghana. 2005. *HIV and AIDS Policy Document*. Accra, Ghana: CCG.

-----. 2008. Background Information. http://www.oikoumene.org/en/member-churches/regions/africa/ghana/ccg.html.

Christian Health Association of Ghana. 2005. *Annual Report*. http://www.chagghana.org/history.htm.

Christiansen, Catrine. 2009. AIDS Work and the Religious Sector in Uganda: Do Church-Based and Faith-Based Aid to AIDS Differ? Paper presented to the Conference of the International Research Network on Religion and AIDS in Africa, Lusaka, Zambia, April 15-17.

Church World Service, Ecumenical Advocacy Alliance, Norwegian Church Aid, UNAIDS, and World Conference of Religions for Peace. 2006. Scaling up Effective Partnerships: A Guide to Working with Faith-Based Organisations in the Response to HIV and AIDS. http://www.e-alliance.ch/media/media-6695.pdf.

Churches Health Association of Zambia. 2005. *Strategic Plan, 2006-2011*. Lusaka: CHAZ.

------. 2009. Impact of HIV/AIDS on Religion. Presentation to the Conference of the International Research Network on Religion and AIDS in Africa, Lusaka, Zambia, April 15-17.

CIDA. *See* Canadian International Development Agency.

Circle of Concerned African Women Theologians. 2002. Sex, Stigma and HIV/AIDS: African Women Challenging Religion, Culture and Social Practices. Report of the Third Pan African Conference, Addis Ababa, Ethiopia, August 4-8. http://www.thecirclecawt.org/annual_report?mode=content&id=17498&refto=2638.

Collier, Paul. 2009. *Wars, Guns and Votes*. New York: Harper.

Cooper, Barbara. 2006. *Evangelical Christians in the Muslim Sahel*. Bloomington: Indiana University Press.

Cox, Harvey. 1968. *The Secular City*. Harmondsworth, UK: Penguin.

Csete, Joanne. 2007. Rhetoric and Reality: HIV/AIDS as a Human Rights Issue. In *The Global Politics of AIDS*, ed. Paul Harris and Patricia Siplon, 247-261. Boulder, CO: Lynne Rienner Publishers.

Czerny, Michael. 2007. ARVs When Possible. In *AIDS in Africa—Theological Reflections*, ed. Bénézet Bujo and Michael Czerny, 97-103. Nairobi: Paulines Publications Africa.

------. 2009. A Human and Spiritual Wake Up Call. *Thinking Faith Jesuit Newsletter*. http://www.thinkingfaith.org/articles/20090325_1.pdf.

Czerny, Michael, and Robert Vitillo. 2005-2006. The Church's Role and Approaches in HIV/AIDS Advocacy. *African Ecclesial Review* 47-48 (4-1): 274-289.

Dahl, Robert. 1956. *A Preface to Democratic Theory*. Chicago: University of Chicago Press.

Davies, Elizabeth. 1983. Correspondent's Report: Africa and the World Council of Churches. *Africa Today* 30 (1/2): 86-88.

DGAAN. *See* DuPage Glocal AIDS Action Network.

Diamond, Larry. 1988. Introduction: Roots of Failure, Seeds of Hope. In *Democracy in Developing Countries: Africa*, ed. Larry Diamond, Juan Linz, and Seymour Martin Lipset, 1-32. Boulder, CO: Lynne Rienner Publishers.

Dilger, Hansjörg. 2007. Healing the Wounds of Modernity: Salvation, Community and Care in a Neo-Pentecostal Church in Dar Es Salaam, Tanzania. *Journal of Religion in Africa* 37 (1): 59-83.

-----. 2010. Heavenly Action: Religion, Class and the "Failures" of AIDS Activism in Urban Tanzania. Paper presented at the AIDS, Religion and Social Activism Workshop, International Research Network on AIDS and Religion in Africa, Makerere University, Kampala, July 6.

Dube, Musa. 2002. Fighting with God: Children and HIV/AIDS in Botswana. *Journal of Theology for Southern Africa* 114 (November): 31-42.

DuPage Glocal AIDS Action Network. 2008. *Keeping the Promise: Leaders in Making Poverty History*. Sixth Annual Report. http://www.dgaan.org/pdfs/2008/2008dgaanreport.pdf.

Ecumenical Advocacy Alliance. n.d. Exploring Solutions: Talking about AIDS with Your Church. http://www.e-alliance.ch/fileadmin/user_upload/docs/EAA_ExploringSolutionsHIVPreventionChurch_A4_EN.pdf.

------. 2005. Framework for Action: The HIV and AIDS Campaign (2005-2008). http://www.e-alliance.ch.

Ecumenical HIV and AIDS Initiative in Africa. 2002. Background Information. http://www.oikoumene.org/en/programmes/justice-diakonia-and-responsibility-for-creation/hivaids-initiative-in-africa-ehaia.html.
EHAIA. *See* Ecumenical HIV and AIDS Initiative in Africa.
Ellis, Stephen, and Gerrie ter Haar. 1998. Religion and Politics in Sub-Saharan Africa. *Journal of Modern African Studies* 36 (2): 175-201.
------. 2004. *Worlds of Power: Religious Thought and Political Practice in Africa*. New York: Oxford University Press.
Ellis, Stephen, and Ineke van Kessel. 2009. *Movers and Shakers: Social Movements in Africa*. Leiden, NL: Brill Publishers.
Emerson, Michael, and Christian Smith. 2000. *Divided by Faith: Evangelical Religion and the Problem of Race in America*. New York: Oxford University Press.
Englebert, Pierre. 2000. *State Legitimacy and Development in Africa*. Boulder, CO: Lynne Rienner Publishers.
------. 2009. *Africa: Unity, Sovereignty and Sorrow*. Boulder, CO: Lynne Rienner Publishers.
Englund, Harri. 2000. The Dead Hand of Human Rights: Contrasting Christianities in Post-Transition Malawi. *Journal of Modern African Studies* 38 (4): 579-603.
------. 2003. Christian Independency and Global Membership: Pentecostal Extraversions in Malawi. *Journal of Religion in Africa* 33 (1): 83-111.
Epstein, Helen. 2005. God and the Fight Against AIDS. *New York Review of Books*. April 25. http://www.nybooks.com/articles/archives/2005/apr/28/god-and-the-fight-against-aids.
------. 2007. *The Invisible Cure: Why We Are Losing the Fight Against AIDS in Africa*. New York: Picador.
Evangelical Presbyterian Church, Ghana. n.d. E. P. Church Policy on HIV/AIDS. Ho, Ghana: EPC.
Ewing, Deborah. 2002. Welfare. In *Impacts and Interventions: The HIV/AIDS Epidemic and the Children of South Africa*, ed. Jeff Gow and Chris Desmond, 79-94. Pietermaritzburg, South Africa: University of Natal Press.
Expanded Church Response. n.d. Factsheet. Lusaka, Zambia: Expanded Church Response.
Farmer, Paul. 2005. *Pathologies of Power: Health, Human Rights, and the New War on the Poor*. Los Angeles: University of California Press.
Fatton, Robert. 1995. Africa in the Age of Democratization: The Civic Limitations of Civil Society. *African Studies Review* 38 (2): 67-110.
FBO Roundtable. 2009. The Role of Religion in Fighting HIV/AIDS in Zambia. Open discussion to the Conference of the International Research Network on Religion and AIDS in Africa, Lusaka, Zambia, April 15-17.
Fenio, Kenly Greer. 2005. Bush's Funding of Religion in Ethiopia through the President's Emergency Plan for AIDS Relief (PEPFAR): HIV/AIDS, the Ethiopian Orthodox Church, and Community Beliefs. Paper presented at the Conference on African Health and Illness, University of Texas-Austin, March 25-27.
------. 2009. Between Bedrooms and Ballots: The Politics of HIV's "Economy of Infection" in Mozambique. Ph.D. diss., University of Florida.
Fikansa, Chanda. 2009. Reflections on the Contradictions of ARVs from a Practitioner Perspective. Paper presented at the Conference of the

International Research Network on Religion and AIDS in Africa, Lusaka, Zambia, April 15-17.
Firmin-Sellers, Kathryn. 1995. The Politics of Property Rights. *American Political Science Review* 89 (4): 867-881.
Fowler, Alan. 1997. *Striking a Balance: A Guide to Enhancing the Effectiveness of Non-Governmental Organizations in International Development.* London: Earthscan.
Freedom House. 2009. Freedom in the World 2009: Table of Independent Countries. http://www.freedomhouse.org/uploads/fiw09/FIW09_Tables&GraphsForWeb.pdf.
Freston, Paul. 2001. *Evangelicals and Politics in Asia, Africa and Latin America.* New York: Cambridge University Press.
Friedman, Steven, and Shauna Mottiar. 2004. A Moral to the Tale: The Treatment Action Campaign and the Politics of HIV/AIDS. Paper for the Centre for Policy Studies. Durban, South Africa: University of KwaZulu-Natal.
Gallup News Service. 2007. *Africans' Confidence in Institutions—Which Country Stands Out?* News Release. http://www.gallup.com/poll/26176/Africans-Confidence-Institutions-Which-Country-Stands-Out.aspx.
Garner, Robert. 2000a. Religion as a Source of Social Change in the New South Africa. *Journal of Religion in Africa* 30 (3): 310-343.
------. 2000b. Safe Sects? Dynamic Religion and AIDS in South Africa. *Journal of Modern African Studies* 38 (1): 41-69.
George, Timothy, Os Guinness, John Huffman, Rich Mouw, Jesse Miranda, David Neff, Richard Ohman, Larry Ross, and Dallas Willard. 2008. *An Evangelical Manifesto.* http://www.anevangelicalmanifesto.com.
Gifford, Paul. 1992. *New Dimensions in African Christianity.* Nairobi, Kenya: All Africa Conference of Churches.
------. 1998. *African Christianity: Its Public Role.* Bloomington: Indiana University Press.
------. 2004. *Ghana's New Christianity: Pentecostalism in a Globalizing African Economy.* Bloomington: Indiana University Press.
------. 2009. *Christianity, Politics and Public Life in Kenya.* New York: Columbia University Press.
Gill, Anthony. 1998. *Rendering unto Caesar: The Catholic Church and the State in Latin America.* Chicago: University of Chicago Press.
Gill, Peter. 2006. *Body Count: Fixing the Blame for the Global AIDS Catastrophe.* New York: Thunder's Mouth Press.
Global Fund to Fight AIDS, Tuberculosis, and Malaria. 2003a. Application for Round 1, Ghana. http://www.theglobalfund.org/programs/grant/?compid=529&grantid=26&lang=en&CountryId=GHN.
------. 2003b. Application for Round 1, Zambia. http://www.theglobalfund.org/grandocuments/1ZAMH_577_82_full.pdf.
------. 2005. Application for Round 4, Zambia. http://www.theglobalfund.org/grandocuments/4ZAMH_831_0_full.pdf.
------. 2006a. Application for Round 5, Ghana. http://www.theglobalfund.org/programs/grant/?compid=1026&grantid=448&lang=en&CountryId=GHN.
------. 2006b. Report on the Involvement of FBOs in the Global Fund. http://www.theglobalfund.org/documents/publications/other/FBOReport/GlobalFund_FBO_Report_en.pdf.

------. 2007. Global Fund Grants Progress. http://www.theglobalfund.org/en/distributionfunding/?lang=en.
------. 2008a. Application for Round 8, Ghana. http://www.theglobalfund.org/programs/grant/?compid=1677&lang=en&CountryId=GHN.
------. 2008b. Application for Round 8, Zambia. http://www.theglobalfund.org/programs/grant/?compid=1781&lang=en&CountryId=ZAM.
------. 2008c. Distribution of Funding after 7 Rounds. http://www.theglobalfund.org/en/distributionfunding/?lang=en.
------. 2009. Background. http://www.theglobalfund.org/en.
------. 2010a. Country Coordinating Mechanisms. http://www.theglobalfund.org/en/ccm/?lang=en.
------. 2010b. Ghana—Grant Portfolio. http://portfolio.theglobalfund.org/Country/Index/GHN?lang=en#.
Global Health Council. 2005. Faith in Action: Examining the Role of Faith-Based Organizations in Addressing HIV/AIDS. http://www.globalhealth.org/view_top.php3?id=448.
Gorter, Karen. 2006. Church Tithes Building Fund. *The Banner* 141 (5): 15.
Gray, Peter. 2004. HIV and Islam: Is HIV Prevalence Lower among Muslims? *Social Science & Medicine* 58 (9): 1751-1757.
Gray, Ronald, David Serwadda, Godfrey Kigozi, Fred Nalugoda, and Maria Wawer. 2006. Uganda's HIV Prevention Success: The Role of Sexual Behavior Change and the National Response. Commentary on Green *et al.* (2006). *AIDS and Behavior* 10 (4): 347-350.
Green, Edward. 2003. *Rethinking AIDS Prevention: Learning from Successes in Developing Countries.* Greenport, CT: Praeger.
Green, Edward, and Allison Ruark. 2008. AIDS and the Churches: Getting the Story Right. *First Things* 182 (April): 22-26.
Gusman, Alessandro. 2009. HIV/AIDS, Pentecostal Churches, and the "Joseph Generation" in Uganda. *Africa Today* 56 (1): 66-86.
Guth, James, Lyman Kellstedt, John Green, and Corwin Smidt. 2001. America Fifty/Fifty. *First Things* 116 (October): 19-26.
------. 2006. Religious Influences in the 2004 Presidential Election. *Presidential Studies Quarterly* 36 (2): 223-242.
Gyimah-Boadi, E. 2004. Civil Society and Democratic Development. In *Democratic Reform in Africa: The Quality of Progress*, ed. E. Gyimah-Boadi, 99-119. Boulder, CO: Lynne Rienner Publishers.
Haddad, Beverley. 2002. Gender Violence and HIV/AIDS: A Deadly Silence in the Church. *Journal of Theology for Southern Africa* 114 (November): 93-106.
------. 2005. Reflections on the Church and HIV/AIDS. *Theology Today* 62 (1): 29-37.
Halbert, Debora, and Christopher May. 2005. AIDS, Pharmaceutical Patents, and the African State. In *The African State and the AIDS Crisis*, ed. Amy S. Patterson, 195-218. Aldershot, UK: Ashgate Publishers.
Harbeson, John, Donald Rothchild, and Naomi Chazan, ed. 1994. *Civil Society and the State in Africa*. Boulder, CO: Lynne Rienner Publishers.
Hasty, Jennifer. 2005. *The Press and Political Culture in Ghana*. Bloomington: Indiana University Press.

Haven, Bernard. 2005. Is Aid for AIDS "Exceptional"? Risk, Dependence and the Good Governance Paradigm. M.S. thesis, London School of Economics.

Haven, Bernard, and Amy S. Patterson. 2007. The Government-NGO Disconnect: AIDS Policy in Ghana. In *The Global Politics of AIDS*, ed. Paul Harris and Patricia Siplon, 65-86. Boulder, CO: Lynne Rienner Publishers.

Haynes, Jeffrey. 2007. *Religion and Development: Conflict or Cooperation?* New York: Palgrave MacMillan.

Haynes, Naomi. 2009. My Wealth, Your Health: Prosperity Theology and the Praxis of Care Among Zambian Pentecostals. Paper presented at the Conference of the International Research Network on Religion and AIDS in Africa, Lusaka, Zambia, April 15-17.

Hearn, Julie. 2002. The Invisible NGO: U.S. Evangelical Mission in Kenya. *Journal of Religion in Africa* 32 (1): 32-60.

Hendriks, Jurgens, and Johannes Erasmus. 2001. Interpreting the New Religious Landscape in Post-Apartheid South Africa. *Journal of Theology of Southern Africa* 109 (March): 41-65.

Heywood, Linda. 2007. The Angolan Church: The Prophetic Tradition, Politics, and the State. In *The Catholic Church and the Nation-State: Comparative Perspectives*, ed. Paul Christopher Manuel, Lawrence Reardon, and Clyde Wilcox, 191-206. Washington, DC: Georgetown University Press.

Hoge, Dean, and Jackson Carroll. 1978. Determinants of Commitment and Participation in Suburban Protestant Churches. *Journal of the Scientific Study of Religion* 17 (2): 107-127.

Human Rights Watch. 2005. *The Less They Know, the Better: Abstinence-Only HIV/AIDS Programs in Uganda*. Report for Human Rights Watch. http://hrw.org/reports/2005/uganda0305.

-----. 2007. Letter to Congressional Caucus about US Support for Ugandan Homophobia. http://www.hrw.org/en/news/2007/10/10/letter-congressional-caucus-about-us-support-ugandan-homophobia.

-----. 2008. Letter to the Uganda Authorities Regarding Recent Arrest of LGBT Activists. http://www.hrw.org/en/news/2008/06/10/letter-ugandan-authorities-regarding-recent-arrest-lgbt-activists.

Hunter, Susan. 2003. *Black Death: AIDS in Africa*. New York: Palgrave MacMillan.

Huntington, Samuel. 1968. *Political Order in Changing Societies*. New Haven, CT: Yale University Press.

------. 1991. *The Third Wave: Democratization in the Late Twentieth Century*. Norman: University of Oklahoma Press.

------. 1996. *The Clash of Civilizations*. New York: Simon and Schuster.

Hyden, Goran. 1980. *Beyond Ujamaa in Tanzania: Underdevelopment and an Uncaptured Peasantry*. Berkeley: University of California Press.

Iliffe, John. 2006. *The African AIDS Epidemic: A History*. Oxford: James Currey.

INERELA+. *See* International Network of Religious Leaders Living with or Personally Affected by HIV and AIDS.

International Network of Religious Leaders Living with or Personally Affected by HIV and AIDS. 2010. Background Information. http://www.inerela.org/english/about-us.

Inter-Religious Council of Uganda. 2010. Unpublished answers to questions for panel debate. Distributed at the AIDS, Religion and Social Activism Workshop, International Research Network on AIDS and Religion in Africa, Makerere University, Kampala, July 8.

------. n.d. HIV Prevention Program. Pamphlet.

IRCU. *See* Inter-Religious Council of Uganda.

Jenkins, Philip. 2007. *The Next Christendom: The Coming of Global Christianity*. New York: Oxford University Press.

Johnson, Krista. 2004. The Politics of AIDS Policy Development and Implementation in Postapartheid South Africa. *Africa Today* 51 (2):107-128.

Joint United Nations Program on HIV/AIDS. 2005a. *AIDS in Africa: Three Scenarios to 2025*. http://data.unaids.org/Publications/IRC-pub07/jc1058-aidsinafrica_en.pdf .

------. 2005b. *Evidence for HIV Decline in Zimbabwe: A Comprehensive Review*. http://data.unaids.org/publications/irc-pub06/ zimbabwe_epi_report_nov05_en.pdf.

------. 2006. *Report on the Global AIDS Epidemic*. http://www.unaids.org/ en/KnowledgeCentre/HIVData/GlobalReport/2006/default.asp.

------. 2007. *UNAIDS and WHO Underline Importance of Evidence Based Approaches to Treatment in Response to AIDS*. Public Statement. http://data.unaids.org/pub/PressStatement/2007/070316_gambia_statement _en.pdf.

------. 2008a. *Ghana Country Progress Report*. http://data.unaids.org/pub/ Report/2008/ghana_2008_country_progress_report_en.pdf.

------. 2008b. *Report on the Global AIDS Epidemic*. http://www.unaids.org/en/ KnowledgeCentre/HIVData/GlobalReport/2008/2008_Global_report.asp.

------. 2008c. *Zambia Country Progress Report. Multi-Sectoral AIDS Response Monitoring and Evaluation Biennial Report*. http://data.unaids.org/pub/ Report/2008/zambia_2008_country_progress_report_en.pdf.

------. 2009a. *AIDS Epidemic Update*. http://data.unaids.org/pub/Report/ 2009/JC1700_Epi_Update_2009_en.pdf.

------. 2009b. *Botswana Country Response*. http://www.unaids.org/en/ CountryResponses/Countries/botswana.asp.

------. 2009c. *Namibia Country Response*. http://www.unaids.org/en/ CountryResponses/Countries/namibia.asp.

------. 2009d. *Rwanda Country Response*. http://www.unaids.org/en/ CountryResponses/Countries/rwanda.asp.

------. 2009e. *Uganda Epidemiological Fact Sheet on HIV and AIDS*. http://apps.who.int/globalatlas/predefinedReports/EFS2008/full/EFS2008_ UG.pdf.

------. 2010a. Greater Involvement of People Living with or Affected by AIDS. Background Statement. http://www.unaids.org/en/PolicyAndPractice/ GIPA/default.asp.

------. 2010b. Young People Are Leading the HIV Prevention Revolution. Report for UNAIDS. http://data.unaids.org/pub/Outlook/2010/ 20100713_outlook_youngpeople_en.pdf.

Joseph, Richard. 1993. The Christian Churches and Democracy in Contemporary Africa. In *Christianity and Democracy in Global Context*, ed. John Witte, 231-247. Boulder, CO: Westview Press.

Joshua, Steve. 2009. Miracles of Care and Treatment: A Historical-Critical Analysis of South African Catholic Responses to HIV/and Aids between 2000 and 2005. Paper presented to the Conference of the International Research Network of Religion and AIDS in Africa, Lusaka, Zambia, April 15-17.

Kaiser Family Foundation. 2009. HIV Testing in the United States. http://www.kff.org/hivaids/upload/6094-09.pdf.

Kaiser Family Foundation and Pew Forum. 2007. *A Global Look at Public Perceptions of Health Problems, Priorities, and Donors: The Kaiser/Pew Global Health Survey*. http://www.kff.org/kaiserpolls/7716.cfm.

Kajubi, Phoebe, Moses Kamya, H. Fisher Raymond, Sanny Chen, George Rutherford, Jeffrey Mandel, and Wili McFarland. 2008. Gay and Bisexual Men in Kampala, Uganda. *AIDS Behavior* 12: 492-504.

Kalipeni, Ezekiel, Adamson Muula, and Olivia Mchaju Liwewe. 2009. HIV and Religion in Africa: The Politics of Treatment and Prevention in a Changing Religious Landscape. Paper presented at the Conference of the International Research Network on Religion and AIDS in Africa, Lusaka, Zambia, April 15-17.

Kalu, Ogbu. 2008. *African Pentecostalism: An Introduction*. New York: Oxford University Press.

Kangale, Chabu. 2009. INERELA+ Dismantling HIV and AIDS Related Stigma and Discrimination. Presentation to the Conference on Mobilizing Religious Health Assets for Transformation, African Religious Health Assets Programme, Cape Town, South Africa, July 13-16.

Kaoma, Kapya. 2010. The U.S. Christian Right and the Attack on Gays in Africa. *Public Eye Magazine* 2 (4). http://www.publiceye.org/magazine/v24n4/us-christian-right-attack-on-gays-in-africa.html.

Kasfir, Nelson, ed. 1998. *Civil Society and Democracy in Africa*. London: Frank Cass.

Katongole, Emmanuel. 2005. *A Future for Africa: Critical Essays in Christian Social Imagination*. Scranton, NJ: University of Scranton Press.

Keck, Margaret, and Kathryn Sikkink. 1998. *Activists Beyond Borders: Advocacy Networks in International Politics*. Ithaca, NY: Cornell University Press.

Kelly, Michael. 2007. The Response of the Christian Churches to HIV/AIDS in Zambia. In *Christian Ethics and HIV/AIDS in Africa*, ed. J. N. Amanze, 185-201. Gaborone, Botswana: Bay Publishing.

------. 2009. Historic View of the Reaction of Churches/Religion Towards Stigmatizing Disease. Presentation at the Conference of the International Research Network on Religion and AIDS in Africa, Lusaka, Zambia, April 15-17.

Kielland, Anne, and Maurizia Tovo. 2006. *Children at Work: Child Labor Practices in Africa*. Boulder, CO: Lynne Rienner Publishers.

Kiirya, Stephen. 1998. *HIV/AIDS in Uganda: A Comprehensive Analysis of the Epidemic and the Response*. Report for Uganda AIDS Commission. http://www.aidsuganda.org/pdf/Status_report_1998.pdf.

Krakauer, Mark. 2004. Churches' Responses to AIDS in Two Communities in KwaZulu-Natal, South Africa. MA thesis, Oxford University. http://siteresources.worldbank.org/DEVDIALOGUE/Resources/ChurchAIDS.pdf.

Krakauer, Mark, and Jodie Newbery. 2007. Churches' Responses to HIV/AIDS in Two South African Communities. *Journal of the International Association of Physicians in AIDS Care* 6 (1): 27-35.

Krasner, Stephen. 1982. Structural Causes and Regime Consequences: Regimes as Intervening Variables. *International Organization* 36 (2): 185-205.

Kwansa, B. K. 2009. The "Spiritual" and Living with HIV/AIDS in Ghana: Negotiations, Compromises and Outright Surrender in Search of Spiritual Therapy. Paper presented at the Conference of the International Research Network on Religion and AIDS in Africa, Lusaka, Zambia, April 15-17.

Lalor, Kevin. 2004. Child Sexual Abuse in Sub-Saharan Africa: A Literature Review. *Child Abuse & Neglect* 28 (4): 439-460.

Lancaster, Carol. 2000. *Transforming Foreign Aid.* Washington, DC: Institute for International Economics.

Little, Eric, and Carolyn Logan. 2008. *The Quality of Democracy and Governance in Africa: New Results from Afrobarometer Round 4.* Working Paper 108. http://www.afrobarometer.org/papers/ AfropaperNo108_21may09_newfinal.pdf.

Longman, Timothy. 2010. *Christianity and Genocide in Rwanda.* New York: Cambridge University Press.

Lubaale, Nicta. 2008. *Community Action on HIV and AIDS.* Church Education Booklet 5, Organization of African Instituted Churches. Oxford: Strategies for Hope Trust.

Lynch, Cecelia. 2010. AIDS Prevention or AIDS Orphans: Faith-Based and Interfaith Interventions in Cameroon and Kenya. Paper presented at the AIDS, Religion and Social Activism Workshop, International Research Network on AIDS and Religion in Africa, Makerere University, Kampala, July 6.

Maluleke, Tinyiko. 2001. The Challenge of HIV/AIDS for Theological Education: Towards an HIV/AIDS Sensitive Curriculum. *Missionalia* 29 (2): 125-143

Mann, Jonathan. 1999. Human Rights and AIDS: The Future of the Pandemic. In *Health and Human Rights: A Reader*, ed. Jonathan Mann, Sofia Gruskin, Michael Grodin, and George Annas, 216-226. New York: Routledge.

Manuel, Paul Christopher, Lawrence Reardon, and Clyde Wilcox, eds. 2007. *The Catholic Church and the Nation-State: Comparative Perspectives.* Washington, DC: Georgetown University Press.

Manuh, Takyiwaa, ed. 2005. *At Home in the World? International Migration and Development in Contemporary Ghana and West Africa.* Accra, Ghana: Sub-Saharan Publishers.

March, James, and Johan Olsen. 1989. *Rediscovering Institutions: The Organizational Basis of Politics.* New York: The Free Press.

Marshall, Katherine. 2001. Development and Religion: A Different Lens on Development Debates. *Peabody Journal of Education* 76 (3-4): 339-375.

------. 2008a. The ABCs of AIDS. *First Things* (August-September): 2-4.

------. 2008b. Faith to the Fore on Malaria. Blog Entry. http://newsweek.washingtonpost.com/onfaith/georgetown/2008/09/faith_to_the_fore_on_malaria.html.

Marshall, Katherine, and Marisa van Saanen. 2007. *Development and Faith: Where Mind, Heart, and Soul Work Together.* Washington, DC: World Bank.

Marshall, Mandy, and Nigel Taylor. 2006. Tackling HIV and AIDS within Faith-Based Communities: Learning from Attitudes on Gender Relations and Sexual Rights within Local Evangelical Churches in Burkina Faso, Zimbabwe, and South Africa. *Gender and Development* 14 (3): 363-374.

Marshall, Thomas. 1964. *Class, Citizenship and Social Development.* New York: Doubleday.

Martin, David. 1990. *Tongues of Fire: The Explosion of Protestantism in Latin America.* Oxford: Blackwell.

Massad, Joseph. 2002. Re-Orienting Desire: The Gay International and the Arab World. *Public Culture* 14 (2): 361-385.

Maxwell, David. 2000. "Catch the Cockerel before Dawn": Pentecostalism and Politics in Post-Colonial Zimbabwe. *Africa: Journal of the International African Institute* 70 (2): 249-277.

McCarthy, John, and Mayer Zald. 1977. Resource Mobilization and Social Movements: A Partial Theory. *American Journal of Sociology* 82 (6): 1212-1241.

Melucci, Alberto. 1996. *Challenging Codes: Collective Action in the Information Age.* New York: Cambridge University Press.

Meyer, Birgit. 1998. Commodities and the Power of Prayer: Pentecostalist Attitudes Towards Consumption in Contemporary Ghana. *Development and Change* 29 (4): 751-776.

------. 2004. Christianity in Africa: From African Independent to Pentecostal-Charismatic Churches. *Annual Review of Anthropology* 33: 447-474.

Mhungu, Samuel. 2007. HIV/AIDS and the Church in Zimbabwe. Presentation to the Conference of the Network for African Congregational Theology, Lusaka, Zambia, August 4-11.

Micah Challenge. n.d. The Micah Challenge: Mobilising Christians Against Poverty. Unpublished leaflet.

Michael, Sarah. 2004. *Undermining Development: The Absence of Power among Local NGOs in Africa.* Bloomington: Indiana University Press.

Miller, Donald, and Tetsunao Yamamori. 2007. *Global Pentecostalism: The New Face of Christian Social Engagement.* Los Angeles: University of California Press.

Mills, Edward, William A. Schabas, Jimmy Volmink, Roderick Walker, Nathan Ford, Elly Katabira, Aranka Anema, Michel Joffres, Pedro Cahn, and Julio Montaner. 2008. Should Active Recruitment of Health Workers from Sub-Saharan Africa Be Viewed as a Crime? *Lancet* 371 (February): 685-688.

Moe, Terry. 1990. Political Institutions: The Neglected Side of the Story. *Journal of Law, Economics, and Organization* 6 (special issue): 213-253.

Monsma, Stephen. 2001. Christian Commitment and Political Life. In *In God We Trust: Religion and American Political Life,* ed. Corwin Smidt, 255-268. Grand Rapids, MI: Baker Academic Publishers.

Morgan, Rosemary. 2010. Religion and the HIV/AIDS Responses of Faith-Based NGOs. Paper presented at the AIDS, Religion and Social Activism Workshop, International Research Network on AIDS and Religion in Africa, Makerere University, Kampala, July 6.

Morgan, Timothy. 2005. Warren, Hybels Urge Churches to Wage 'War on AIDS.' *Christianity Today Magazine.* December 5. http://www.christianitytoday.com/ct/2005/decemberweb-only/12.0.html.

Moss, Todd. 2007. *African Development: Making Sense of the Issues and Actors*. Boulder, CO: Lynne Rienner Publishers.

Msoka, Colman. 2009. Religion and AIDS in Africa: Christian Construction of ARVs. Paper presented at the Conference of the International Research Network on Religion and AIDS in Africa, Lusaka, Zambia, April 15-17.

Mugambi, J. N. K. 1996. African Churches in Social Transformation. *Journal of International Affairs* 50 (Summer): 193-220.

Mukonyora, Isabel. 2008. Foundations for Democracy in Zimbabwean Evangelical Christianity. In *Evangelical Christianity and Democracy in Africa*, ed. Terence Ranger, 131-160. New York: Oxford University Press.

Mukuka, Lawrence, and Vered Slonim-Nevo. 2006. The Role of the Church in the Fight Against HIV/AIDS Infection in Zambia. *International Social Work* 49 (5): 641-649.

Mwenda, Andrew. 2004. What Are Museveni's Numbers on Third Term? *Monitor Publications*. http://www.mail-archive.com/ugandanet@kym.net/msg11115.html.

Myandawire, Thandika, and Charles Souldo. 1999. *Our Continent, Our Future: African Perspectives on Structural Adjustment*. Trenton, NJ: Africa World Press.

Nabalonzi, J. K. 2000. Empowering Children and Communities on Child Sexual Abuse and HIV/AIDS. Paper presented at the International Conference on AIDS, Durban, South Africa, July 9-14. Abstract MoPeE2863.

NAC. *See* National HIV/AIDS/STI/TB Council.

National HIV/AIDS/STI/TB Council. 2005. *Zambia Country Report*. http://data.unaids.org/pub/Report/2006/2006_country_progress_report_zambia_en.pdf?preview=true.

Ndhlovu, Japhet. 2007. Combating HIV: A Ministerial Strategy for Zambian Churches. Ph.D. diss., Stellenbosch University, South Africa.

NETACT. *See* Network for African Congregational Theology.

Network for African Congregational Theology. n.d. Synopsis of Goals and Protocol. Unpublished document.

Newell, Jonathan. 1995. 'A Moment of Truth'? The Church and Political Change in Malawi, 1992. *Journal of Modern African Studies* 33 (2): 243-262.

North, Douglass. 1990. *Institutions, Institutional Change and Economic Performance*. New York: Cambridge University Press.

Northmead Assembly of God. 2009. Information. http://www.northmead assembly.org

Okaalet, Peter. 2002. The Role of Faith Based Organizations in the Fight against HIV and AIDS in Africa. *Transformation* 19 (4): 274-278.

Omenyo, Cephas. 2008. African Christian Initiatives: Some Lessons for the West. Byker Chair Presentation at Calvin College, Grand Rapids, MI, May 6.

Ondetti, Gabriel. 2006. Repression, Opportunity, and Protest: Explaining the Takeoff of Brazil's Landless Movement. *Latin American Politics and Society* 48 (2): 61-94.

Oppong, Christine, M. Yaa P.A. Oppong, and Irene K. Odotei, eds. 2006. *Sex and Gender in an Era of AIDS*. Accra, Ghana: Sub-Saharan Publishers.

Oppong, Joseph, and Samuel Agyei-Mensah. 2004. HIV/AIDS in West Africa: The Case of Senegal, Ghana, and Nigeria. In *HIV & AIDS in Africa:*

Beyond Epidemiology, ed. Ezekiel Kalipeni, Susan Craddock, Joseph Oppong, and Jayati Ghosh, 70-81. Malden, MA: Blackwell Publishing.

Overa, Ragnhild. 2007. When Men Do Women's Work: Structural Adjustment, Unemployment and Changing Gender Relations in the Informal Economy of Accra, Ghana. *Journal of Modern African Studies* 45 (4): 539-563.

Overberg, Kenneth. n.d. What Does the Church Say About HIV/AIDS? *National Catholic AIDS Network Newsletter*. http://www.ncan.org/resources/church_say.cfm.

Parry, Sue. 2003. *Responses of Faith-Based Organisations to HIV/AIDS in Sub Saharan Africa*. http://www.wcc-coe.org/wcc/what/mission/fba-hiv-aids.pdf.

Paterson, Gillian. 2001. *AIDS and African Churches: Exploring the Challenges*. London: Christian Aid.

------. 2009. HIV Prevention: A Global Theological Conversation. http://www.e-alliance.ch/fileadmin/user_upload/docs/EAA_HIVPreventionGlobalTheologicalConversation_Intro_EN.pdf.

Patterson, Amy S. 1998. A Reappraisal of Democracy in Civil Society: Evidence from Rural Senegal. *Journal of Modern African Studies* 36 (3): 423-441.

------. 1999. The Dynamic Nature of Citizenship and Participation: Lessons from Three Rural Senegalese Cases. *Africa Today* 46 (1): 3-28.

------. 2003. The Institutions of Senegalese Development Organizations. *African Studies Review* 46 (3): 35-54.

------. 2006. *The Politics of AIDS in Africa*. Boulder, CO: Lynne Rienner Publishers.

------. 2009. Developing Countries: HIV/AIDS as a Human Rights Issue. *Encyclopedia of Human Rights*, ed. David Forsythe, 26-36. London: Oxford University Press.

Patterson, Amy S., and Dave Cieminis. 2005. Weak and Ineffective? African States and Recent International AIDS Policies. In *The African State and the AIDS Crisis*, ed. Amy S. Patterson, 171-193. Aldershot, UK: Ashgate Publishers.

Patterson, Eric. 2005. Religious Activity and Political Participation: The Brazilian and Chilean Cases. *Latin American Politics and Society* 46 (4): 1-29.

Paul B. Henry Institute. 2009. The Disappearing "God Gap" in American Politics. *Newsletter* 10 (Summer): 1-2.

PEPFAR. *See* US President's Emergency Plan for AIDS Relief.

Pew Forum. 2006. Spirit and Power: A 10-Country Survey of Pentecostals. http://www.pewforum.org/surveys/pentecostal/africa.

------. 2008. Global Anglicanism at a Crossroads. Report. http://pewforum.org/docs/?DocID=309.

------. 2010. Tolerance and Tension: Islam and Christianity in Sub-Saharan Africa. Report. http://pewforum.org/uploadedFiles/Topics/Belief_and_Practices/sub-saharan-africa-preface.pdf.

Pew Global Attitudes Project. 2002. U.S. Stands Alone in Its Embrace of Religion. Press Release. http://www.people-press.org.

Pfeiffer, James. 2004. Condom Social Marketing, Pentecostalism, and Structural Adjustment in Mozambique: A Clash of AIDS Prevention Messages. *Medical Anthropology Quarterly* 18 (1): 77-103.

Philpott, Daniel. 2004. The Catholic Wave. *Journal of Democracy* 15 (2): 32-46.
------. 2007. Explaining the Political Ambivalence of Religion. *American Political Science Review* 101 (3): 505-526.
Phiri, Isaac. 2000. Proclaiming Peace and Love: A New Role for Churches in African Politics. *Journal of Church and State* 42 (4): 781-802.
------. 2001. *Proclaiming Political Pluralism: Churches and Political Transitions in Africa*. Westport, CT: Praeger.
PMI. *See* US President's Malaria Initiative.
Pobee, John. 1991. *Religion and Politics in Ghana*. Accra, Ghana: Asempa Publishers.
Poku, Nana, and Alan Whiteside. 2004. *The Political Economy of AIDS in Africa*. Aldershot, UK: Ashgate Publishers.
Potts, Malcolm, Daniel Halperin, Douglas Kirby, Ann Swidler, Elliot Marseille, Jeffrey Klausner, Norman Hearst, Richard Wamai, James Kahn, and Julia Walsh. 2008. Reassessing HIV Prevention. *Science* 320 (May): 749-750.
Powder, Jackie. 2006. Targeting Persistent Killers. *Johns Hopkins Public Health Online Magazine*. http://magazine.jhsph.edu/2006/Spring/africa/news/child_health.
Presbyterian Church of Ghana. 2002. *AIDS Policy Statement*. Accra, Ghana: PCG.
Putnam, Robert. 1994. *Making Democracy Work*. Princeton, NJ: Princeton University Press.
Putzel, James. 2004. The Global Fight Against AIDS: How Adequate Are the National Commissions? *Journal of International Development* 16 (8): 1129-1140.
Ranger, Terence, ed. 2008. *Evangelical Christianity and Democracy in Africa*. New York: Oxford University Press.
Rasmussen, Louise. 2009. Catholic Involvement with ART in Uganda—Negotiating Ideals of Holistic Care with Therapeutic Citizenship. Paper presented at the Conference of the International Research Network on Religion and AIDS in Africa, Lusaka, Zambia, April 15-17.
Rice, Andrew. 2004. Enemy's Enemy. *The New Republic* 231 (6): 18-21.
Riddell, Roger C. 2008. *Does Foreign Aid Really Work?* Oxford: Oxford University Press.
Roll Back Malaria. 2009. Background. http://www.rollbackmalaria.org.
Root, Robin. 2009. Being Positive in Church: Religious Participation and HIV Disclosure Rationale Among People Living with HIV/AIDS in Rural Swaziland. *African Journal of AIDS Research* 8 (3): 295-309.
Rosberg, Carl, and Robert Jackson. 1982. *Personal Rule in Black Africa*. Berkeley: University of California Press.
Rutagambwa, Elisée. 2007. The Rwandan Church: The Challenge of Reconciliation. In *The Catholic Church and the Nation-State: Comparative Perspectives*, ed. Paul Christopher Manuel, Lawrence Reardon, and Clyde Wilcox, 173-190. Washington, DC: Georgetown University Press.
Sackey, Brigid. 2006. *New Directions in Gender and Religion: The Changing Status of Women in African Independent Churches*. Lanham, MD: Lexington Books.

Sambo, Boubacar, Michelle Fraser, and Souleymane Issoufou. 2008. Study of Activities and Needs in the Field of HIV/AIDS in Niger. Report for Christian Reformed World Relief Committee, Grand Rapids, Michigan.

Schaffer, Frederic. 1998. *Democracy in Translation: Understanding Politics in an Unfamiliar Culture*. Ithaca, NY: Cornell University Press.

Schmid, Barbara. 2006. AIDS Discourses in the Church: What We Say and What We Do. *Journal of Theology of Southern Africa* 125 (July): 91-103.

Scott, James. 1976. *The Moral Economy of the Peasant*. New Haven, CT: Yale University Press.

Šehović, Annamarie Bindenagel. 2010. Development Dependence: Assuming Responsibility. *Consultancy Africa Intelligence*. February 15. http://www.consultancyafrica.com/index.php?option=com_content&view=article&id=348:development-dependence-assuming-responsibility&catid=61:hiv-aids-discussion-papers&Itemid=268.

Seidel, Gill. 1993. The Competing Discourses of HIV/AIDS in Sub-Saharan Africa: Discourses of Rights and Empowerment vs Discourses of Control and Exclusion. *Social Science & Medicine* 36 (3): 175-194.

Siegle, Joseph, Michael Weinstein, and Morton Halperin. 2004. Why Democracies Excel. *Foreign Affairs* 83 (5): 57-71.

Simpson, Anthony. 2009. *Boys to Men in the Shadow of AIDS: Masculinities and HIV Risk in Zambia*. New York: Palgrave MacMillan.

Siplon, Patricia. 2002. *AIDS and the Policy Struggle in the United States*. Washington, DC: Georgetown University Press.

-----. 2010. Can Faith and Rights-Based Movements Be Allies in the Fight Against HIV/AIDS? Lessons from North America and Africa. Paper presented at the AIDS, Religion and Social Activism Workshop, International Research Network on AIDS and Religion in Africa, Makerere University, Kampala, July 8.

Skillen, James. 2004. *Pursuit of Justice: Christian-Democratic Explorations*. Lanham, MD: Rowman Littlefield.

Smith, Raymond, and Patricia Siplon. 2006. *Drugs into Bodies*. Westport, CT: Praeger.

Snow, David, E. Burke Rochford, Steven Worden, and Robert Benford. 1986. Frame Alignment Processes, Micromobilization, and Movement Participation. *American Sociological Review* 51 (4): 464-481.

South African Presbyterian Church. 2009. Organizational Information. http://users.iafrica.com/d/da/danman/history.html.

Ssempa, Martin. 2005. Testimony before the Full Committee on "US Response to the Global AIDS Crisis: A Two Year Review." US House Committee on International Relations, Rayburn House Office Building, Washington, DC, April 13.

------. 2009. Personal Background. http://www.martinssempa.com.

------. 2010. Ugandan Pastors' Response to Rick Warren over the Anti-Homosexuality Bill 2009. http://www.martinssempa.com/warren-response.html.

Stiglitz, J. 2006. *Making Globalization Work: The Next Steps to Global Justice*. London: Allen Lane.

Stillwaggon, Eileen. 2006. *AIDS and the Ecology of Poverty*. New York: Oxford University Press.

Stryker, Sheldon, Timothy Owens, and Robert White, eds. 2000. *Self, Identity, and Social Movements*. Minneapolis: University of Minnesota Press.

Supreme Pontiff Paul VI. 1968. *Humanae Vitae*. Encyclical Letter, Rome, July 25. http://www.vatican.va/holy_father/paul_vi/encyclicals/documents/hf_p-vi_enc_25071968_humanae-vitae_en.html.

Tarrow, Sidney. 1989. *Democracy and Disorder: Protest and Politics in Italy 1965-1975*. Oxford: Clarendon Press.

Thomas, Scott. 2005. *The Global Resurgence of Religion and the Transformation of International Relations*. New York: Palgrave MacMillan.

Tippett, Krista. 2008. Evangelical Politics: Three Generations. Radio Program on *Speaking of Faith*, American Public Media, April 17.

Tripp, Aili Mari. 1997. *Changing the Rules: The Politics of Liberalization and the Urban Informal Economy in Tanzania*. Berkeley: University of California Press.

Truman, David. 1951. *The Governmental Process*. New York: Alfred Knopf.

UCSF. *See* University of California, San Francisco.

Uganda Religious Leaders. 2010. Panel Debate at the AIDS, Religion and Social Activism Workshop, International Research Network on AIDS and Religion in Africa, Makerere University, Kampala, July 7.

UNAIDS. *See* Joint United Nations Program on HIV/AIDS.

UNDP. *See* United Nations Development Program.

UNICEF. *See* United Nations Children's Fund.

United Nations. 2000. Millennium Development Goals: End Poverty by 2015. http://www.un.org/millenniumgoals/bkgd.shtml.

------. 2001. *Declaration of Commitment on HIV/AIDS*. http://www.un.org/ga/aids/docs/aress262.pdf.

United Nations Children's Fund. 2009a. Diarrhoea: Why Children Are Still Dying and What Can Be Done. http://www.who.int/child_adolescent_health/documents/9789241598415/en/index.html.

------. 2009b. Maternal Mortality Fact Sheet. www.unicef.org/specialsession/about/sgreport-pdf/09_MaternalMortality_D7341Insert_English.pdf.

------. 2010. Statistics by Area: Child Protection. http://www.childinfo.org/discipline.html?q=printme.

United Nations Development Program. 2005. *Human Development Report*. New York: United Nations.

University of California, San Francisco. 2008. *What Works Best in HIV Prevention Globally?* Report for the Center for AIDS Prevention Studies. http://www.caps.ucsf.edu/pubs/FS/international.php.

------. 2009. *President's Emergency Plan for AIDS Relief (PEPFAR): An Overview*. http://hivinsite.ucsf.edu/InSite?page=pr-rr-10.

Upendo Village. 2009. Background Information. http://www.upendovillage.org.

US Agency for International Development. 2008. Ghana: HIV/AIDS Health Profile. http://www.usaid.gov/missions/gh.

US Assemblies of God. 2009. Background Information. http://ag.org/top/About/structure.cfm.

US Department of State. Bureau of Democracy, Human Rights and Labor. 2008a. *International Religious Freedom Report 2008*. http://www.state.gov/g/drl/rls/irf/2008/index.htm.

------. 2008b. *Zimbabwe: International Religious Freedom Report 2008*.

http://www.state.gov/g/drl/rls/irf/2008/108399.htm.
US President's Emergency Plan for AIDS Relief. 2006. New Partners Initiative. http://www.pepfar.gov/c19532.htm.
------. 2007. US President's Emergency Plan for AIDS Relief Partners. http://www.pepfar.gov/partners.
US President's Malaria Initiative. 2009. Saving Lives in Africa. http://www.fightingmalaria.gov.
USAID. *See* US Agency for International Development.
Uvin, Peter. 1998. *Aiding Violence: The Development Enterprise in Rwanda*. West Hartford, CT: Kumarian Press.
van de Walle, Nicolas. 2001. *African Economies and the Politics of Permanent Crisis*. New York: Cambridge University Press.
van Stekelenburg, Jacqueline, and Bert Klandermans. 2009. Social Movement Theory: Past, Present and Prospects. In *Movers and Shakers: Social Movements in Africa*, ed. Stephen Ellis and Ineke van Kessel, 17-43. Leiden, NL: Brill Publishers.
Vanden, Harry, and Gary Prevost. 2006. *Politics of Latin America: The Power Game*. New York: Oxford University Press.
Vander Meulen, Rebecca. 2010. Activism in the Diocese of Niassa: Preliminary Observations on Motivating Factors. Paper presented at the AIDS, Religion and Social Activism Workshop, International Research Network on AIDS and Religion in Africa, Makerere University, Kampala, July 6.
Ver Beek, Kurt Alan. 2006. The Impact of Short-Term Missions: A Case Study of House Construction in Honduras after Hurricane Mitch. *Missiology: An International Review* 34 (4): 477-495.
Verba, Sidney, Kay Schlozman, and Henry Brady. 1995. *Voice and Equality*. Cambridge, MA: Harvard University Press.
Villalón, Leonardo. 1995. *Islamic Society and State Power in Senegal*. New York: Cambridge University Press.
VonDoepp, Peter. 1998. The Kingdom Beyond *Zasintha*: Churches and Political Life in Malawi's Post-Authoritarian Era. In *Democratization in Malawi: A Stocktaking*, ed. Kings Phiri and Kenneth Ross, 102-126. Blantyre, Malawi: Christian Literature Association in Malawi.
Walshe, Peter. 1997. Christianity and the Anti-Apartheid Struggle: The Prophetic Voice within Divided Churches. In *Christianity in South Africa: A Political, Social and Cultural History*, ed. Richard Elphick and T. R. H. Davenport, 383-399. Berkeley: University of California Press.
WARC. *See* World Alliance of Reformed Churches.
Warner, Carolyn, and Manfred Wenner. 2006. Religion and the Political Organization of Muslims in Europe. *Perspectives on Politics* 4 (3): 457-479.
Watt, Melissa, Suzanne Maman, Mark Jacobson, and John Laiser. 2009. Missed Opportunities for Religious Organizations to Support People Living with HIV/AIDS: Findings from Tanzania. *AIDS Patient Care and STDs* 23 (5): 389-394.
WCC. *See* World Council of Churches.
WEA. *See* World Evangelical Alliance.
Weigel, George. 1992. *The Final Revolution: The Resistance Church and the Collapse of Communism*. Oxford: Oxford University Press.

Welch, Claude. 2001. Mobilizing Morality: The World Council of Churches and Its Program to Combat Racism, 1969-1994. *Human Rights Quarterly* 23 (4): 863-910.

West, Gerald. 2003. Reading the Bible in the Light of HIV/AIDS in South Africa. *Ecumenical Review* 55 (4): 335-344.

Wheaton College. 2008. Defining Evangelicals and Fundamentalists. http://www.wheaton.edu/isae/defining_evangelicalism.html.

Whiteside, Alan. 2005. The Economic, Social, and Political Drivers of the AIDS Epidemic in Swaziland: A Case Study. In *The African State and the AIDS Crisis*, ed. Amy S. Patterson, 97-126. Aldershot, UK: Ashgate Publishers.

WHO. *See* World Health Organization.

Wilson, David. 2006. HIV Epidemiology: A Review of Recent Trends and Lessons. http://data.unaids.org/pub/ExternalDocument/2007/20060913wilson_en.pdf.

Wolterstorff, Nicholas. 2008. *Justice: Rights and Wrongs*. Princeton, NJ: Princeton University Press.

Woodrow Wilson International Center for Scholars. 2005. *Challenges and Change in Uganda*. Summary of papers presented at Conference on Uganda: An African "Success" Past Its Prime? http://www.wilsoncenter.org/topics/pubs/Uganda1.pdf.

World Alliance of Reformed Churches. 2004. *Covenanting for Justice in the Economy and the Earth* (The Accra Confession). http://warc.jalb.de/warcajsp/news_file/doc-159-1.pdf.

------. 2009. More about WARC. http://warc.jalb.de/warcajsp/side.jsp?news_id=2&part2_id=19&navi=8.

World Assemblies of God Fellowship. 2009. Background. http://www.agcongress.org/01_abot/abt_agfellowship.html.

World Council of Churches. 2000. New Instrument for Global Advocacy: Founding Meeting of the Ecumenical Advocacy Alliance. http://www.wcc-coe.org/wcc/news/press/00/38pre.html.

------. 2001. Increased Partnership between Faith-Based Organizations, Government and Inter-Governmental Organisations. Statement by Faith-Based Organizations, UN General Assembly Special Session on HIV/AIDS, New York, June 25-27. http://www.wcc-coe.org/wcc/what/mission/ny-statement.html.

-----. 2005a. *Healing Mission of the Church*. Preparatory Paper 11. http://www.oikoumene.org/resources/documents/wcc-commissions/mission-and-evangelism/cwme-world-conference-athens-2005/preparatory-paper-n-11-the-healing-mission-of-the-church.html.

------. 2005b. *Working with People Living with HIV/AIDS Organizations*. Report for World Council of Churches. http://www.oikoumene.org/en/resources/documents/wcc-programmes/justice-diakonia-and-responsibility-for-creation/health-and-healing/hivaids/wcc-statements-and-studies/2005-working-with-people-living-with-hivaids-organizations.html.

------. 2009. Who Are We? http://www.oikoumene.org/en/who-are-we.html.

------. 2010. Member Churches. http://www.oikoumene.org/en/member-churches.html.

World Evangelical Alliance. 2009. About Us. http://www.worldevangelicals.org/aboutwea.

World Health Organization. 2000. *Effectiveness of Male Latex Condoms in Protecting Against Pregnancy and Sexually Transmitted Infections*. Fact Sheet 243. http://www.who.int/mediacentre/factsheets/fs243/en.

------. 2005. Zambia: Summary Country Profile for HIV/AIDS. http://www.who.int/hiv/HIVCP_ZMB.pdf.

------. 2007. Faith-Based Organizations Play a Major Role in HIV/AIDS Care and Treatment in Sub-Saharan Africa. http://www.who.int/mediacentre/news/notes/2007/np05/en.

World Vision. 2009. World Vision's Pastors Vision Trips. http://www.worldvision.org/content.nsf/getinvolved/c2c-pastors-vision-trips.

Yirenkyi, Kwasi. 2000. The Role of the Christian Churches in National Politics: Reflections from Laity and Clergy in Ghana. *Sociology of Religion* 61 (3): 325-338.

Youde, Jeremy. 2007. *AIDS, South Africa and the Politics of Knowledge.* Aldershot, UK: Ashgate Publishers.

Zambian Government. 2002. *Demographic Health Survey*. Lusaka, Zambia: Central Statistical Office.

Index

About the Book

Situating her analysis squarely within the context of debates about the role of religion in African politics and society, Amy Patterson systematically analyzes the efforts (and sometimes lack of effort) of Christian churches in shaping HIV/AIDS policy.

Patterson considers how theological worldviews, material resources, historical interactions with the state, and global networks influence church advocacy on AIDS. She is particularly interested in why various churches have responded in such differing ways to the political questions associated with the AIDS epidemic. With the issue of AIDS as a focal point, she offers a cross-national, critical analysis of Christian church mobilization in Africa.

Amy S. Patterson is associate professor of political science at Calvin College. She is author of *The Politics of AIDS in Africa* and editor of *The African State and the AIDS Crisis*.